Swara Yoga

Copyright © Yoga Satsanga Ashram UK 2020

Written by
Yogachariya Jnandev
Yogachariya Dr Ananda Balayogi Bhavanani

Editor & Illustrator
Yogacharini Deepika Saini

ISBN 978-1-9995850-8-2

First Published July 2020

Designed, Printed & Published by Design Marque

Printed in Great Britain by www.designmarque.co.uk

Preface

I offer my gratitude to all the great yogis and the Gurus who have experienced and taught these amazing teachings of swara yoga. I would especially like to thank the masters of the Rishiculture Ashtanga Yoga linaege, Swami Gitananda Giri, Ammaji Meenakshi Devi Bhavanani and Dr Ananda Balayogi Bhavanani.

It has been a real pleasure to produce this Book under the mentorship of my Guru Yogachariya Dr Ananda Balayogi Bhavanani. He has guidance and input has been invaluable and also its a great honour to have him as a Co author. My sincere Pranams to him and the lineage.

This book would not have come to fruition without the help of my Divine wife and our three beautiful boys inspiring me every moment. I am very appreciative of the artwork by Yogacharini Deepika since she has recently taken this on it has given a new dimension for our yoga work together with her artwork from a yoga practitioners view of inner experience or vision.

I have been following Swara yoga for many years from the Nath and Giri traditions, and always found the practices and teachings inspiring, balancing and transformative in my own health wellbeing and transcendental experiences. I was first initiated into Swara yoga in 2001 by Swami Balaknath in Rajasthan and given the book on Shiva Swarodaya by Charandas ji Maharaj, which I found very insightful and mystic text. Since then I have always been curious about understanding these ideas from our modern perspective. In recent years reading some of the Bihar school of Yogas work and Dr Ananda Balayogi Bhavananis therapeutic research work on Swara yoga has added the fuel of inspiration in my soul to do this work.

Since my own intense sadhana using these Swara yoga practices I really believe that with the study and sincere practice of swara yoga we can bring huge transformation to bring about holistic health, wellbeing and spiritual evolution. For those who crave transcendental or yogic experiences then the swara yoga practices can be a great aid to this. In the therapeutic sense one can experience great benefits even by changing the swaras 4-5 times a day for several weeks. I give all my good wishes to the true Yoga seekers and hope this book can assist many of you.

Blessings

Yogachariya Jnandev (Surender Saini) and Yogacharini Deepika (Sally Saini) are an integral part of my Gitananda Yoga family worldwide and I am so proud of the way they have been able to develop through hard work the Yoga Satsanga Ashram in Carmarthenshire, Wales and well as their new International Ashram developing in Portugal. Having visited their Ashram in Wales, I can vouch for the beautiful spiritual ambiance that can be felt there and it is a joy to teach in such a Yogic atmosphere.

May the Guru Parampara continue to bless Yogachariya Jnandev, Yogacharini Deepika and their family as well as the Yoga family of the Yoga Satsanga Ashram with success in their Sadhana.

My dear Yogachemmal Jnandev has come out with this excellent book that takes a detailed view of the Swara Yoga concepts of the Indian Yoga tradition. These are teachings that bring together the Yogic and Tantric perspectives as they deal with the universal energies that are flowing through us through the medium of the all important breath.

The modern equivalent of Swara is the nasal cycle which is an ultradian rhythm of nasal congestion and decongestion with a quasi-periodicity of 60 to 240 minutes. Though Keyser made the first formal description and the use of the term nasal cycle in 1895, this concept and an understanding of its role in human life had existed for much longer in Indian thought. The Vedic science dealing with nasal cycle and its functions was known as Swarodaya Vigjnan (swara = sonorous sound produced by airflow through nostrils, udaya = functionality, and vigjnan = knowledge).

Shivaswarodaya, is an ancient Sanskrit treatise that gives us immense guidance in this field of yogaadvises us to undertake quieter, passive activities (soumya karya) when left nostril flow is dominant (ida / chandra swara), engage in challenging and exertional activities (roudra karya) when right nostril is dominant (pingala / surya swara) and to relax or meditate when bilateral nasal flow is operational (sushumna swara). Ida swara (left nostril dominance) is described as feminine, Shakti and moon-like (chandra) while pingala swara (right nostril dominance) is described as masculine, Shiva and sun-like (surya).

In fact the traditional Indian cultural iconographic description of Lord Shiva as Ardhanarishwara has Shakti (femininity) depicted as the left half of the body while Shiva (masculinity) is the right half. Such notion of left-right, female-male duality is common in oriental traditional medicine as also in western alchemy.

I wish that this book serves as a noble guide for all dedicated and sincere students and practitioners of Yoga who wish to expand their perspective of Yoga beyond just Asana. Those who wake up in consciousness and realize that, "what we know is just a handful, what we have to yet learn is infinite like the Universe".

May we all grow and glow in spirit through the life of Yoga, enabling each and every one to manifest their inherent divinity with joy, health and wellness.

Om Hari Om tat Sat Om.

Yogacharya Dr Ananda Balayogi Bhavanani

MBBS, MD(AM), C-IAYT, DSc (Yoga)

Director and Professor of Yoga Therapy, CYTER of Sri Balaji Vidyapeeth and Chairman

ICYER at Ananda Ashram, Pondicherry, India. www.icyer.com

Contents:

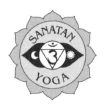

Swara Yoga

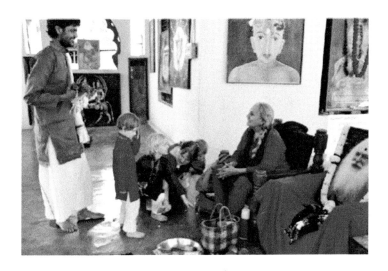

Swara Yoga : The Importance of Guru

In the modern age, teachings and practices are easily available to everyone through our books, media, and internet. Nowadays you will find lectures on every subject on YouTube, and many other audio-video resources. Still to learn and follow some of these Yogic Sciences and practices, it is advisable to find a competent Guru, teacher or guide. You Guru or teacher is not only going to guide you through the practices, but also help you understanding your own self and prepare for these practices.

Most of these ancient teachings and scriptures were written in the last few thousands years on stones, leaves, barks and slates made from clay or stone. So their Kriyas and Prakriyas were written in a codified and condensed form. Its almost like bullet points or reminders when you go out for an important meeting.

Ancient Yoga teachings for thousands years passed down in Guru-Shishya Paramapara (from teacher to student) in a typical Ashram or Gurukula system by word of mouth. These Gurus of masters would examine and prepare the students for years through Karma Yoga, Bhakti Yoga, Jnana Yoga, and Hatha Yoga for years before some of these advance teachings will take place. A Guru will wait or search for Adhikari - a student who is ready and eligible to learn and master the teachings to be passed down.

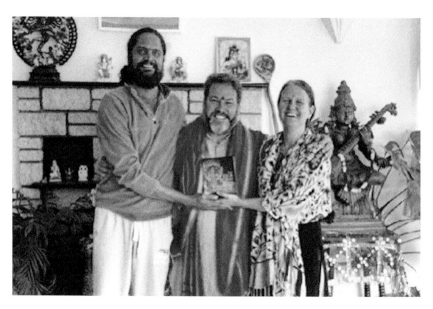

Guru is a Sanskrit term for master or guide, which literally translates as "one who leads us from darkness to light" or "one who dispels the darkness of ignorance". So it is important to find a Guru, as well as develop the right attitude and will to learn and master these divine teachings. Without the attitude of service or Seva, Sraddha or faith, Samarpan or devotion, Tapas or dedicated practice, there is not fruit or success on the path of Yoga Sadhana.

In India, even now, there is immense respect, faith and understanding of the Guru-Shishya concept. Due to so many of the modern spiritual Gurus or masters taking advantage of their position and power, this divine concept and relationship of Guru and Shishya has been questioned worldwide.

As the stress levels and toxicity in life is growing at physical, mental, emotional, energetic and spiritual levels, Yoga, especially Hatha Yoga, has been followed worldwide and becoming more and more popular each day.

I personally here will advise you to find a Guru or teacher to learn Hatha Yoga, Pranayama, Raja Yoga, Mantra Yoga, and Swara yoga for success in your Sadhana. In particular, the Swara Yoga, Kundalini Yoga and Samayama are some of the advanced and inner Sadhana Paths and you will need a guide who can help you prepare and guide your spiritual journey.

The Shiva Samhita (3:9) mentions: "Having received instructions in Yoga, and followed guidance of a guru who has experienced Yoga, let him (student or follower also known as Sadhaka) practice with sincerity according to the method taught by the teacher for spiritual success."

These Kriyas and Prakriyas are very powerful and can lead us to spiritual experiences and are kept secret as they can also cause disturbances to our physical, mental and emotional balance. These practices develop an immense amount of Pranic and energy and we don't know how to channel them or utilise them, these energies can be also destructive in nature. Remember energy is not constructive or destructive. Energy only becomes useful if it being used to the benefit of human evolution and the same energy can be used to destroy lives.

Guru-Shisya (The TEACHER and Disciple)

To understand life and grow on the path of yoga and spirituality, vairagya [non-attachment] and abhyasa [practices] are the responsibility of the Sadhaka/seeker. When these two are truly undertaken, another help follows or comes in the form of Guru and Grace, each inter-linked, each so beautiful, eternal and joyful, each so intense and powerful. Unfortunately, most frequently each are misunderstood!

Western culture, which has increasingly welcomed and embraced traditions from the East, often understood Guru to mean simply a Teacher. In the West Guru is generally considered to be a spiritual master; yoga or meditation master; or a master of philosophy. The Guru is expected to share his wisdom and experiences and help his followers or disciples to attain the state of liberation or mastery in one or other field of life. The Guru is the one who passes the wisdom, experiences and blessings he/she has experienced as has been passed on to them by their masters, rather than just the information or knowledge.

In ancient times in India education was carried out in guru-kulas/ ashrams. The shisyas/ students have to live with their Guru from an early age and were given not only instruction on an intellectual level, but also were guided in spiritual development and in the maintenance of physical health. The Guru had a very close relationship with the students and knew their habits and levels of inner strength.

The word Guru is a compound of two root words, Gu and Ru. Gu means darkness and Ru means light. That which dispels the darkness of ignorance is called Guru. The energy and action of removing darkness are Guru. Guru is not a person, it is a force driven by grace. Guru is one who guides you, motivates you to keep moving on the right yoga path.

One of the famous Indian poets says that "the Guru and God both are standing here to whom I should salute first. The God says that I should be grateful to my Guru has guided me on this path to God-realisation." Here importance is given to the Guru as he is the one who has guided the disciple to come that far. Keep in mind that the Guru is one who guides and initiates into the spiritual and yoga practices. By power of sadhana/ practice the sadhaka can achieved the higher states of yoga. The Guru is the one who instruct about practices, motivates in the moments a disciple needs it. The Guru can seem to be harsh and painful in the moments when breaking our ego and getting us out of mental conditions and our comfort zone.

There tend to be a moments in everyone's life where we human beings desire to experience the higher self, God and approach one or other Spiritual disciplines. Everyone's desire or thirst will vary.

It depends on development of vairajna/ non-detachment and abhyasa/ practice. The Guru is always there with and within but the sadhaka /seeker may not be ready to receive, and absorb, learn, practice and experience what the Guru has to offer. You can realise, see or perceive your Guru only when you are ready to receive the higher message.

Many times we even tend to ignore or neglect our Guru because of Samsaya/doubt in the Guru or our own self. The Guru introduces you to the practices and instructs or guides you how to go on for your own journey. The Guru introduces you to the teaching you are ready to follow. Many times we might have doubt that our Guru is not teaching us, or introducing us to the higher practices.

In India Guru is a sacred word that is used with reverence and is always associated with the highest wisdom. The Guru is unique in a person's life. The relationship between shisya/ disciple and the Guru is like no other relationship. It is said that the guru is not mother, father, son, or daughter. The guru is not a friend in any conventional sense. It also is sometimes said that the guru is father, mother, son, daughter, and friend all in one; the guru is sun and moon, sky and earth to the disciple.

The relationship of Guru to Shisya/disciple is indescribable. The relationship extends to the realm beyond the world, transcends death, and seen far beyond the limited karmic bonds associated with family and friends. A mother and father help sustain the body of their child, and nurture and guide the child through the formative years of life to adulthood. Guru sustains, nurtures, and guides a soul through lifetimes to attain Samadhi, oneness, self-realisation, liberation.

The relationship with the Guru must be based on the purest form of unconditional love. There should be complete openness with the Guru. The disciple should hold nothing back from the Guru. The disciple goes to the Guru with full faith and entrusts his whole life to his Guru. The Guru accepts his disciple's life and chops it and burns what is not necessary, and then carefully carves what remains into something sacred. When the disciple is ready the Guru sends them back to the world to fulfil all the worldly duties/karmas. The disciple offers his/ her support to the Guru all through his/her life. When the disciples are ready then the Guru authorises them to teach or guide other sadhakas on the path.

As gratitude or respect the disciple always states his/her Lineage of Gurus/ the guru-shisya- paramaparai where from he/she has received the teaching. Teaching or instructing yoga saying its 'my yoga', 'my teachings' or not referring to our Gurus is breaching the Yamas the first step of yoga.

I remembered an incidence when I was living with one of the Gurus in Sariska forest hills, Rajasthan. One of his shisya/disciples used to come there every morning with his cows, offer milk and other dairy products to the Guru and sat around him all the day. The cows used to go around grazing themselves and return back in the afternoon when he had to go back to his family. One day the Guru suddenly opened his eyes after long hours of meditation and shouted at the shepherd to go and take care of his cows. The Guru said he is here to guide him to the path of liberation and not to protect his cows from wild animals. He had enough. Later on I realised that the Guru is not to help us in all our stupid worldly problems, or miseries, but he is the one to show us the path to liberation. Still we have to walk on the path by ourselves.

In your spiritual growth your Guru is not an easy one to deal with. The Guru constantly keeps testing you, puts you in difficult situations with obstacles. In the beginning of your spiritual life everything seems to be harder, intense and painful. This is the process of cleansing as well as awareness. Your Guru helps you to realise all the bitter truths of your own self. Once you let go and surrender to your Guru then your Sadhana will become fruitful and blissful.

Guru is not a physical existence or experience, and guru is not a sensory experience. It is a divine experience. When one allows herself or himself to become a channel for receiving and transmitting the divine knowledge, accessing the astral knowledge and higher consciousness and transferring the same to his disciples, then it happens. The guru manifests. A human being must learn to be selfless, must learn to love. Real and higher love expects nothing. Selfless love is foundation of their enlightenment, and attunes them as channels of knowledge.

The Guru is not the goal. The Guru never wants you to worship him or praise him. The Guru is like a boat for crossing the river. The boat brings you across the river. When the river is crossed the boat is no longer necessary. You shouldn't hang onto the boat after completing the journey, and you certainly don't worship the boat.

Many students come to the Guru with preconceived ideas about the Guru, what he should be like, how he should behave and treat students. They come with their own expectations. Students think or have expectations about what the guru should be teaching. Your Guru gives you or teaches what you need as well as what you deserve or are ready to learn. Guru is not there to teach what you want. Guru is to help you to come out of that comfort zone, which may be painful in the beginning.

Again your faith and trust in the Guru can be your strength to go through. Try not to be upset or stressed in the situations when your Guru is not behaving or treating you in a way you are expecting with your preconception or conditioning. Allow your Guru to guide you, all you need to do is follow the practices, let go of all your preconceptions and conditions as well as expectations. The divine Guru will manifest in you.

A yoga seeker should not worry about who the Guru is, or what the Guru will teach, or what the Guru is like. The yoga seeker's first concern should be preparing himself, organising his life, body and thoughts in a spiritually healthy way, and then working toward a way of life that simplifies and purifies.

Once you meet with the guru, the practices and the way Guru behaves should not be the sadhaka's concern. The sadhaka's work is to act and follow on the instructions and teachings of the Guru, and at the same time, work toward more and more selflessness, and surrender of the ego. These can be difficult attitudes to cultivate for the western mind however as these deeply respectful relationships are not part of western culture.

A spiritual Guru's ways of teaching are multi-faceted and sometimes mysterious. His teachings will have multi-meanings and different senses in every situation. Out of the Guru's teaching a student gets what s/he is ready for. A same savitri rhythm of breathing can be a tool for relaxation, pranayama, and gradually pratya-hara / sensory withdrawal, dharana and meditation.

A great Yogi and spiritual Master Swami Rama says that "The guru does not operate from what seems fair, or outwardly appropriate. He is not constrained by such cultural amenities. He can seem harsh, even brutal. He will put students in situations that make no sense, or are very uncomfortable. He will say things that won't make any sense for months. He will ask things of students that students think are impossible. Everything the guru is doing is for the growth of the student. The student need only have faith in that fact. The guru also teaches without words or actions. As the disciple learns to surrender and move the ego out of the way, and grows more selfless, the ability to learn intuitively from the guru grows."

Swara Yoga

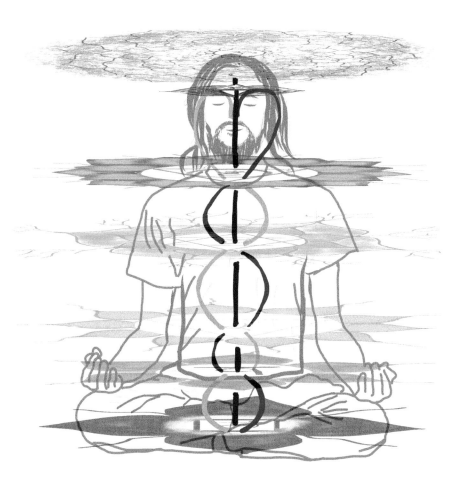

The Swara Yoga teachings come from "Shiva Swarodaya," an ancient Sanskrit Tantric text. This scripture or teachings are in the form of a dialogue between Lord Shiva and his wife Parvati. The text describes that Swara Yoga is useful for the transformation of our life and knowing how to perform various life activities based on breath, nostril and energy.

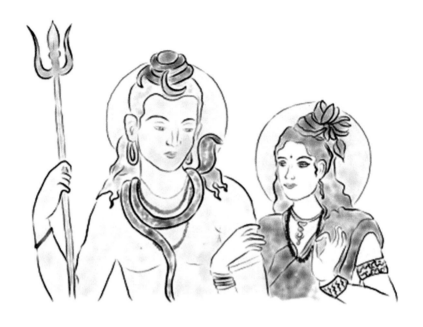

The Swara Yoga teachings were first taught by Lord Shiva to his wife and disciple Parvati. He mentions that in all seven Lokas or planes of consciousness, "He (Shiva) knew no greater wisdom or treasure than Swara Yoga." Here Shiva is the Guru, one dispels the darkness and represents the pure, cosmic and divine consciousness while Parvati represents individual Jiva or consciousness. Inhalation of Puraka is perceived as Parvati or Shakti, when creative potential energies transform in life forces in each life and exhalation is seen as Shiva, or divine consciousness, where Shakti transcending and merging back to cosmic Shiva Consciousness. Through awareness of Swaras or breath one can attain oneness or union of Shiva-Shakti or Individual and Cosmic consciousness.

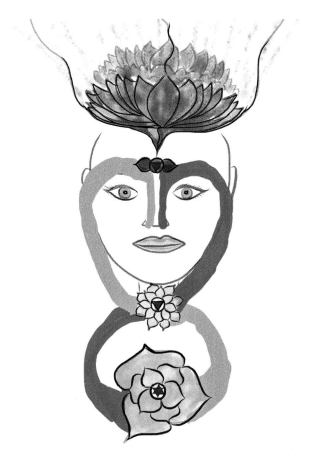

Swara Yoga is the science of breath and prana or life force and explains three Swaras or breathing patterns or modes.

These Swaras are also connected with our prana energy flow and nadis. These are:

1. Ida nadi — breathing dominantly through the left nostril.
2. Pingala nadi — breathing dominantly through the right nostril.
3. Sushumna nadi — breathing through both nostrils.

Once we understand the connection of Swaras with Nadis, body parts, and Chakras, Swara Yoga can provide us many healing practices. In Swara Yoga it is described that the first symptom of any physical and or mental problem can be seen is disturbance in biorhythmic change in nostrils.

Left Nostril : Ida Nadi

This in summary flows in the Left side of the body and is controlled by the Right Brain. This is also known as the feminine and creative principle.

When the breath flows through the left nostril it is known as Ida, or Chandra or the lunar channel. This energy flows down the left side of the spinal cord, and stimulates the right side of the brain. It is symbolically represented by the Chandra or moon, and by the feminine aspect of energy known as Shakti. Ida Swara dominant breathing activates the Parasympathetic nervous system, and hence leads us in good relaxation, healing, and rejuvenation. This also activates effortless flow of creative forces.

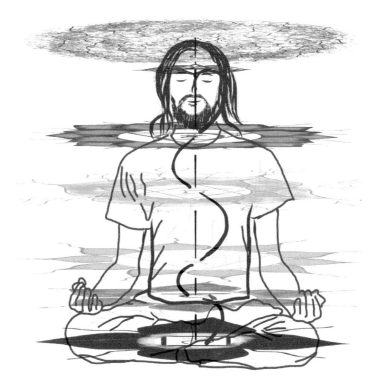

Right Nostril: Pingala Nadi

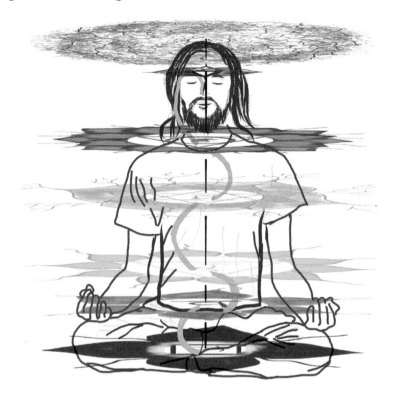

This in summary flows in the Right side of the body, and controls the Left Brain. This is known as masculine and analytical principle.

The right nostril breath is known as Pingala, and is Suriya or the solar channel. This Swara or breath is heating in nature, and is associated with the masculine energy of Shiva. When we inhale through the right nostril, or more accurately when the breath is dominant through this channel it activates the left side of our brain. This is the part of our brain which is associated with our Sympathetic Nervous System.

Swara Yoga - Essence Of The Breath

Swara Yoga is one of the many branches of Yoga of which little has been revealed in Yoga world. The word 'swa' means one's own self, while 'swara' means the breath and relates to the sound of the breath. Therefore, Swara Yoga is the science of breath, prana and self-realisation.

We might ask, why breath is so important in the spiritual evolutionary journey? Not only in Yoga but many other traditions explain that during breathing, divine cosmic energies are drawn into the body. in Yoga we have the terms like SOHAM which relates to the sound of inhalation with SA meaning DIVINE and the exhalation with HAM (pronounced hung) means I. So inhalation in Sanskrita and Yoga is known as Puraka- meaning inhaling the divine life force and exhalation is known as Rechaka – meaning exhaling the I, or ego-self. It is quite similar to the concept of Inspiro-expiro means inhaling the divine spirit and exhaling the darkness.

Here breath becomes the link between individual and cosmic energy and consciousness. With inhalation we are drawing the universal potential prana or conscious energy in our body, which is sustaining all our physical, mental, emotional and spiritual activities. In exhalation we are breathing out individual conscious pranic energy. This represents a perfect balance between Individual and Cosmic Prana, the gross and subtle realms of existence. Tantric teachings explain that whatever exists in the macrocosm exists in the microcosm. This means "we are in this universe and the universe is within us" in a simpler language. So, our individual body is the model of the cosmic body, and the breath is the mediator between the two.

Swara Yoga Scriptures explain that awareness and manipulation of the breath and subtle Pranic energy flow in Nadis will bring balance of body-mind and lead our consciousness into the transcendental realms and ultimately to Samadhi or enlightenment. This science of Swara Yoga explains the significance, principals and concepts of this subtle energy pulsing through various Nadis and the body. Further Swara Yoga details how to regulate, control and utilise our breath, nostrils, Swaras and Nadis to live our life in perfect harmony with nature and biorhythms. In this Sadhana path, breath is the primary tool. When we live in perfect harmony in every aspect, our life and each event becomes effortless. You can think about how effortless plants grow, flowers blossom, birds fly etc.

The Philosophical significance of the breath

The Tantra and Yoga Scriptures as well as Upanishads mention that the subtle life creative force known as Prana and the consciousness are absorbed into the Pranamaya Kosha, then transformed by Chakras flows into your body, primarily, by means of inspiration.

Our breath is referred to as the vehicle of the cosmic energy Prana, Shiva, or Brahman in the Taittriya, Brahamana and Maitri Upanishads.

The Prashna-Upanishad (Ch. 3) states that: "Prana springs from the Atman and is as inseparable from the self as a shadow from its own object or source."

The Bible (Gen. 2 :10) mentions: "And the Supreme God formed man of the dust of the earth and put breathing into his nostrils, the breath of life, he became a living soul. " This means that our physical body has been given consciousness and energy through the breath. The breath itself, being imparted by the cosmic self, thus contains the cosmic force.

In Hinduism and Samkhya it is believed that Atman or the soul is eternal, it doesn't have a beginning and end, it has no birth or death. Atman just exist as the potential conscious energy in the universe. The word death or dead are not commonly used words for people when they die in India. The more commonly used phrases are:- "soul has departed the body", "Prana has left the body", "Last breath has left the body". Here breath is associated with life, prana and the soul and their journey in each and every life form.

Further it explains that each and every life has been given a certain number of breaths. When we complete the number of breaths we are born with, our soul departs from the body. It is a very interesting phenomena as when we relate the breathing pattern, rhythm and frequency, we can easily correlate with the life span of various species. The ancient Yogis recognised that the rate of breath had a correlation with health, state of mind and length of life. Animals that breathe faster have a shorter life span. For example, dogs breathe at a rate of 20-30 times per minute and can live for 10-20 years. The tortoise breathes at a rate of 4 times per minute and lives up to 150 years. Lower the breath rate, higher the life span. We humans breathe at a rate of about 15 times per minute which gives us around 100 years life span. Many Yogis lived for a much longer span by regulating and slowing their breath rate.

Similarly Taoism mentions that "by focusing our mind on the breath, the cosmic divine or creative forces can be experienced within the body. By developing awareness of the breath rather than on coarse sensory objects, ones consciousness and mind can be purified and empowered. Thus, the consciousness is able to transcend from lower levels to higher levels leading from material experiences to higher or cosmic experiences and self-realisation."

According to Scriptures on Pranayama and Swara Yoga, if we can know our breath, we will know the Prana. Once we know the Prana, the knowledge of the whole universe or cosmos can be known. Hence Yogis and Swara Yoga masters mentions that a Sadhaka should work on developing breath awareness, analyse the breath, Swara or Nostril and understand the significance or changes in the body-mind-prana system.

It is mentioned that our breath carries both Prana (vital energy) and Chitta (consciousness) and the force of these energies and their vibration produce the sound.

The Yoga Chudamani Upanishad (V. 31-33) states that: "The exhalation produces the sound HAM and inhalation produces the sound of SO or SA. The Jiva or Soul is continuously repeating the mantra HAMSA 21,000 times, twenty-four hours a day with our Swasha-Praswhas or breathing. This is known as Ajapa Japa." If one silently focuses the mind to his own breath, he will hear the sound of HAMSA or SOHAM. The wisdom of Upanishads mentions that undisturbed awareness of this Japa on the sound of the breath can free Sadhaka from all karmas and lead to absolute liberation. Hence philosophically the breath and power of Swara is very significant from the health and spiritual point of views (Drishti).

Our Breath and Life Span

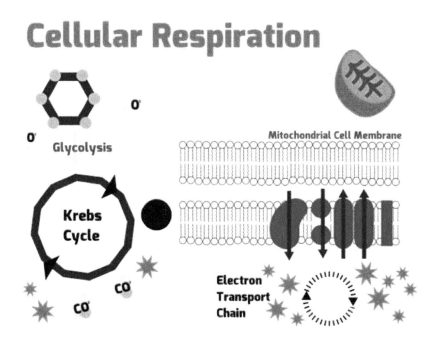

Cellular Respiration

O'
O'
Glycolysis

Krebs Cycle

CO'
CO'

Mitochondrial Cell Membrane

Electron Transport Chain

The great masters of Swara Yoga not only analysed the breath and its relation to the flow of three Nadis and Swaras, but also studied and detailed the nature and quality of breath in correspondence to life span and quality of life. An average healthy person breathes 15 times per minute, 900 times per hour and 21,600 times per day. These Swara Yoga masters explain that each life has been allocated a certain number of breaths in each birth. These numbers of breath are prerecorded in our body corresponding to our Samaskaras and Karmic lessons. If our life span is predetermined by the number of breaths then by slowing down our breath rate, we can enhance not only the quality but also the length of our lifespan.

Some of our recent neuro-physiological research states that the unconscious breathing process in governed by the instinctive and primitive area of the brain, which is situated in the lower cortex area. Our conscious breathing is governed by the higher brain in the upper cortex in the region behind the forehead. When our breathing is conscious and the upper fields of the cortex are active, our breath is slower, rhythmic and deeper. You can easily experience how your breath becomes slower, and relaxed in just a few minutes when you try to focus your mind to your own breath. Our number breaths for each birth are recorded in our lower brain for life survival. All the conscious breaths are not part of this accounting of number of breaths according to spiritual traditions. Also shorter and unconscious breath is laboured and energy consuming and hence adversely effecting quality and quantity of life.

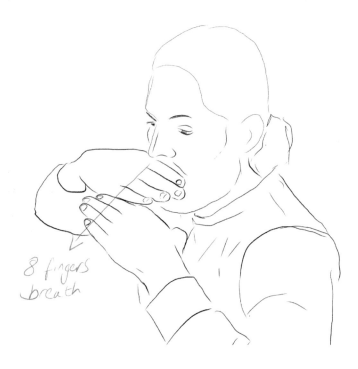

8 fingers
breath

The Swara Yoga teaches us to continuously analyse the nature of the breath and Swara and develop breath awareness or Swash Sakshi Bhava also known as Vipasana of breath. Krishna in Bhagavatd Gita mentions to Arjuna to focus his mind on the tip of his and nose and be aware of each inhalation and exhalation to attain peace and equanimity of mind.

We can easily also notice that each exhalation has a particular length. Yoga texts mention that a normal healthy persons exhalation is of 10 fingers or 7 inches in length.

While mentally or emotionally excited this length of exhalation extends to 12 fingers; while singing this expands to 16 fingers; while eating this expands to 20 fingers; during walking it expands to 24 fingers; sleeping this expands to 30. During states of emotional excitation, the length of exhalation extends to 12 fingers; while singing, 16 fingers; vomiting, 18 fingers; eating, 20 fingers; walking, 24 fingers; sleeping, 30 fingers; and sexual activities it expands up to 36 fingers.

Some scriptures mention that decreasing the length of exhalation will help enhance the vital force and lifespan. Pranayama Yoga teaches us many practices around retention and slower exhalation practices to enhance the Pranic energy. When this Prana energy is enhanced in quantity and quality, it awakens our potential Kundalini and relaxes and rejuvenate our nervous system and awakens all the latent areas of the brain. This brings many Yogic Siddhis and super-natural powers.

Prana – Eternal and All Pervading Cosmic Force

All the Ancient Yogic, Tantra and Upanishads texts refer to the eternally subtle and vital life force known as Prana. This is described as being similar in nature to light. The whole universe exists solely due to this Prana, its primordial force behind all living and non-living beings in this universe. Prana is all pervading. Prana exists in all living and non-living materials but it is neither of all those. Prana is contained in the breath as part of Swara, but it is not the breath.

Prana regulates all organic life as a catalytic force. Like we stored power in a battery in our car to use for starting the engine, it is essential for living organisms to store the Pranic energy to enable all life activities and mobility. By means of Swara Yoga practices access to and storing of this Pranic energy is enhanced and increased, which activates all the latent areas of the nervous system, chakras, and healing systems we are born with. Swara Yoga deals with refining, enhancing and redirecting of this healing Prana to regulate our psycho-physiological health and well-being.

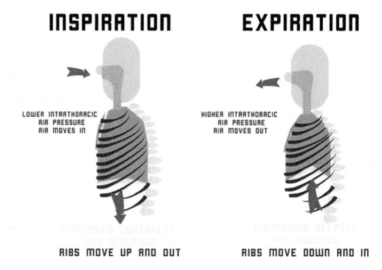

INSPIRATION — LOWER INTRATHORACIC AIR PRESSURE AIR MOVES IN — RIBS MOVE UP AND OUT

EXPIRATION — HIGHER INTRATHORACIC AIR PRESSURE AIR MOVES OUT — RIBS MOVE DOWN AND IN

In last few decades, many renowned scientists have been working on understanding the nature and healing powers of this Pranic energy. Now the subtle aura and energy fields produced by living and non-living materials can be measured or pictured. Prana is the subtlest of catalytic electro-magnetic conscious force. Let's try to look into some modern concepts and ideas to understand Prana and Swara Yoga concepts in context with modern science.

Electromagnetic fields and ions.

It is observed that Pranic transmission can be found in the electromagnetic fields emanating from and throughout the body. Modern scientists describe this energy as a type of bio-energy or bio-electricity. In the 18th century, Luigi Galvani observed the existence of energy fields when he wired up a frog's leg to two conducting rods, and witnessed the energy that pulsated between them. Discovery of Kirlian photography has enabled scientists to actually see the aura or these energetic fields.

Now we all are aware of electric currents flowing through electric wires and magnetic force in electric motors. We somewhat also know how we are harnessing wind power in wind turbines for producing electricity. Primarily, energy is inherent in all materials and our atmosphere, which our geophysicists are exploring in many ways. Ancient Tantra and Yoga masters of Swara Yoga developed the science of understanding and harnessing the subtlest of energy principle.

Our quantum science explains the laws of energy conservation and details quanta as the subtlest form of energy which can be produced, or broken, and it is the primordial force behind the evolution of our universe and life. In this idea we can correlate the word QUANTA with PRANA as it is also said about Prana by great masters and Rishis of Yoga that "Prana is eternal, all-pervading, has no beginning and no end, is always conserved."

Here as in Yoga and Tantra we talk about aura, Pranamaya Kosha or the energetic field in and around the body. Further it mentions that we are a small model of the whole universe. Our earth also has similar electromagnetic and atmospheric fields in and around it.

Earth's magnetic field, also known as the geomagnetic field, is the magnetic field that extends from the Earth's interior out into space, where it interacts with the solar wind, a stream of charged particles emanating from the Sun. Similarly, our bio-energy field also interacts with the cosmic or universal bio-energy field. As our space scientists are exploring outer space, they are noticing various electromagnetic fields charged in atmospheres of various planets, as well as the interconnection between our planets, solar system and beyond. They are proving the findings on inter and intra-relatedness of each and every object, planets, stars, and galaxies.

The Tantra mentions this in a simple godly language Sanskrita as "Yat pinde tat brahmande". This literally means "All that is outside us is within us too," or "Our body is a mini model of the universe." In Sanskrit the word Pinda means "microcosm" and Brahmanda means "macrocosm". So this verse can also be translated as "Whatever is in the microcosm is also in the macrocosm."

These energy fields consist of positively and negatively charged fragments of molecules known as ions. Our life depends on these positive and negative ions for producing life energy. A negative ion has the charge of one electron. A positive ion has the charge of one proton. The Negative ions are the most active electrically between the two.

Negative ions are produced by solar radiations in the upper layers of the atmosphere and are attracted towards the earth by positive ions. During their descent they get trapped by oxygen or nitrogen particles and thereby also charge them with this potential life force. As we breathe, there are many Prana Nadis and their ends are like our nerve endings at cellular level, where these charged particles release this trapped energy. Our cells are automatically energised by the electrical charges of these ions in this process.

Our geoscientists explain the earth as an enormous magnet, generating electromagnetic fields from its opposite poles. The northern and eastern hemispheres are positively charged while the southern and western hemispheres are negatively charged with these ions. These fields both attract and repulse ions in and around the earth, causing a current of movement around the terrestrial plane. Our body also represent the similar energetic fields like the earth and in recent decades science has found ways to measure these currents and energy fields in our body as one organism as well as individually in various parts of our body.

Positive and negative poles

Our body also contains, or produces, its own electromagnetic properties and can be divided into two opposite poles. The Tantra and Yoga texts correlate the upper part of the body with positive or north pole and the lower part of the body with negative or south pole. The right side and back parts of our body are dominated by positive ions while the left side and frontal parts are dominated by negative poles.

Yogis detail the concept of Prana entering through the left side, especially the left hand, and the right side of the body expelling the energy. In therapeutic Pranic healing practices left hand is used are the receiver or absorber of the cosmic energy and the right hand is used as the giver or transfer of this same force. An American theosophical journal illustrated that a ten year old boy from Minnesota developed definite magnetic qualities in his body. The doctors were amazed to witness lightweight metallic objects attracted to his left side, and in particular to his left hand, while the right side of his body remained unaffected.

Swara Yoga practices are based on these positive and negative charges of energy. The Great Rishis describe the negative flow of energy as Ida and the positive flow of energy as Pingala. Modern technology and science has developed many ways to control, manipulate and produce these ions or energies. Most of our machines are working on these principles.

The Great Yogis and Rishis learned and mastered many techniques, kriyas and prakriyas, asanas and mudras, pranayamas and jnana yoga kriyas to channel this bio-energy also, known as Pranas throughout the whole body or a particular point like the Chakra or focus point. The Rishis learned how to connect with cosmic Prana or energy and channel that into individual Pranic energy. The energy always moves higher charged points to the lesser charged points in order to create a balance between negative and positive energy poles.

Swara Yoga teaches us how to manipulate the flow of breath through the nostrils, thereby controlling and changing the energy flows or currents in our own body which regulate the flow of positive and negative currents.
It is by balancing these two poles of energy that the yogi becomes free from two opposite forces causing duality. This brings the awakening of kundalini, which illuminates the fabulous, unexplored areas of the brain and consciousness responsible for all of humanities ingenuity, higher knowledge and self-realisation.

Yoga Polarity in the Gitananda Tradition of Yoga
(From Yoga Step by Step course by Swamiji Gitananda Giri Ji)

Polarity is a term often used in Adhyatmika Yoga, the higher aspect of Yoga, to describe a state where the Yogi is ready for the ultimate Yogic experience of being merged into the oneness or Ultimate Reality. Polarity is described in Physics as the possession by a body of two poles at either extremity of a line of direction passing through a mass, the properties at one pole being of opposite or contrasting nature to the properties at the other end of the pole. Polarity can describe the condition of a magnet, or electromagnetic light waves, or as by transmission through variously oriented crystals or other suitable media or in electricity, or by change in the potential of a cell due to the accumulation of liberated gases. In cellular life, polarisation is by a process of biological ionisation All of these processes lead to a condition of possessing polarity. so that the negative force is able to flow towards its positive counterpart. Union or Yoga takes place.

Yoga or Union cannot take place without there being polarity. A neutral state of harmony. Equilibrium and balance may have value in itself, but only when a powerful "negative flow" joins with an equally powerful "positive base" is true Union possible, This has been the earliest teachings of Yoga. Where Shakta/Shakti—Female/Male Union was contemplated as the ideal to produce enlightenment and Samadhi, Cosmic Consciousness. This energy flow is best described by the Sanskrit term Loma/Viloma, the Process in Yoga of polarising. Loma/Viloma is a Yogic way of expressing a more complicated Sanskrit term "Dhruvabhisaranashila", which actually is more scientifically associated with the description of the polarity of this planet earth. The magnetic energy of this earth flows over the surface of the planet from the north pole to the south pole and through the centre from the south pole to the north pole. A similar polarity Is observed in the human cell in its living function. Polarity Is a description of living, de-polarity, a stale of dying, while electrolysis is death. Electrolysis produces chemical decomposition by electrical changes in the cell. Electrolyte balance Is the normal state in which the action and reaction of two or more electrolyses is of normally balanced proportions.

An electrical charge moving in cellular liquid works upon the mineral elements of the cell. These elements are described as ions. and their balance ionisation, ions such as sodium. Potassium and magnesium move in and out of cells and it is apparent that their movements are not a consequence of free passive diffusion, but by some electrical force producing biological change. These, ions are not in a state of equilibrium, but exist In a "Steady state away from equilibrium" which is referred to by the general term of "active transport". There are a handful of theories in science to explain these electrical changes referred to as the "earlier hypothesis", but these are difficult to understand even in the most simplified explanations.

Yet, the whole process of polarity is the basis of biological and spiritual evolution. For a working theory you need a little knowledge of chemistry, physics and electronics and the necessary vocabulary. This vocabulary must include the terms anion and cation. These two terms are equal to loma/viloma in Sanskrit. Although Loma/Viloma can also mean "more". A single anion contains the smallest amount of energy that exists. Be careful not to mix up the term anion with an atom. A single anion contains one MH unit of energy. But, it may contain as many as 399 MH units of energy. The word anion is both singular and plural. An anion molecule has a positive ion as its nucleus. This positive ion is known as a cation. A single cation contains 503 MH units of energy, but may contain as many as 999 MH units. The anion is the element which in electrolysis passes towards the anode of the positive pole. The cation, the electropositive element that itself moves towards the cathode.

The orbiting shell of an anion molecule rotates in a clockwise direction. Each cation molecule has an anion as its nucleus and has cationic electrons on its outer orbit, which move counter clockwise. Energy is created by the resistance generated when these oppositely charged ions rotating in opposite directions come together. In the world of mass, resistance consumes energy. In the world of energy, resistance creates higher energy. Anion - cation balance is measured as PH in chemistry, but may be measured as resistance of any value.

In Sanskrit the word "Anu" can describe a molecule, while "Paramanu", describes an atom. Loma/Viloma describes the play of energy from anode - cathode. To follow through in electronics, one merely needs an electron tube, a diode permitting electrons to pass in one direction only from the cathode to the anode. This would produce in the Yogic concept a mono-pole magnetic particle or force described as arousal through Sushumna Nadi of Kundalini Shakti in Tantra and Yoga.

Recently, science announced the possible discovery of a monopole magnetic particle. Most magnetised objects are 'dipole' even if separated into the tiniest segments, like a magnet. The monopole would be the counterpart of the positive proton or negative electron that exist independently in nature. The charge on a positron was estimated of 68.5 times as strong as that of a charged electron, or some multiple of 68.5. The positron later proved to have a charge of 137. Physicists have searched for the elusive monopole in everything from ocean from floor minerals to meteorites and moon rocks. It has not yet occurred to them to research the Kundalini phenomenon of Yoga. But at this point, we are interested in something much less than the total Yogic experience, yet producing basic ingredients of Yogic polarity. Yoga practices of Loma-Viloma are the key to this power and its positive control.

Loma Viloma Prakiryas in Gitananda Tradition

Many Asanas can be done as a Loma-Viloma practice. Such postures would have to be grouped where the spinal currents of Ida and Pingala are forced to move downwards or upwards, according to the posture. Dharmika Asana is a Loma flow position, where energy moves upwards from the base of the spine, towards the cranium.

Supta VajraAsana is Viloma position, where the energy moves downwards toward the Kanda at the base of the spine. One may note that the above two postures represent a bending forward and then a bending backwards position typically described as Loma-Viloma. Loma Viloma can be described as convex -concave, as in optic lenses, and when the term is used in Pranayama Yoga, it means converse and inverse breathing.

Loma Pranayama is a three-part breath sometimes described as Visama Vritta Pranayama. The breath is taken in, held in and then let out. Viloma Pranayama is the opposite. The breath is taken in then out, and then held out. The value of the practice is multiple. In Loma Pranayama the blood temperature rises slightly, destroying impurities in the blood. In Viloma Pranayama, the blood temperature falls, reducing the incidence of blood fever. Simple "in and out" breath is termed Sukha Pranayama. If all four parts of breath are done consecutively, that is, in, held in, out, held out, then it is termed Sukha Purvaka Pranayama.

Loma-Viloma Pranayama

Loma-Viloma Pranayama is Alternate Nostril Breathing. The breath begins on an in breath through the right nostril, briefly held in, then released through the left nostril, and briefly held out. A hand gesture called Vishnu Mudra or a comparable gesture called Nasarga Mudra is used to control the alternate nostril flow. The breathing cycle is in the rhythmic pattern of Savitri Pranayama of a : 4 : 8 : 4. This form of Pranavama is called Nadi Shuddni by some Yoga teachers. But it is also called Pratiloma Pranayama by others.

Aloma- Viloma Pranayama

Aloma-Viloma Pranayama is a breath cycle where the incoming breath is on the right nostril. The breath is then let out through the left nostril and then taken in again through the left nostril. The breath is then let out and in again on the right nostril. This cycle is repeated many times, to the pattern Savitri 8 : 4 : 8 : 4. This form of Pranayama actually feeds the nervous system with Prana and is extremely beneficial to those who suffer from neurasthenia and psych-asthenia the most common nerve and emotional condition in the world today. Typified by lassitude, inertia, fatigue and loss of initiative. The psychic state of psych-asthenia is restless fleeting, hypersensitivity, and undue irritability with outburst of tantrums and senseless outrage.

Pratiloma Pranayama

The reverse of the breath pattern is called Pratiloma Pranayama. The breath in Pratiloma Pranayama begins on the left nostril and is taken in and out of the left nostril before shifting over to the right nostril where the same in and out cycle is performed. The entire pattern is repeated many times in a split-rhythm pattern of taking the breath in for a four count, and letting it out for an eight count, Different counts can be used, 5 by 10, 6 by 12 etc.

One yoga school teaches that Pratiloma is Pranayama is to take the breath in through alternate nostrils while breath the is let out through both nostrils. Such a practice is actually the reverse of Surya Bhedana Pranayama and therefore called Chandra Bhedana.

Surya Bhedana Pranayama is also known as Pingala Pranayama, while Chandra Bhedana Pranayama is known as Ida Pranayama.

Anu-Loma -Viloma

A group of Pranayamas which are more than Pranayamas and called Anu-Loma-Viloma and Alu-Loma-Viloma Kriyas are taught in both the Jnana Yoga and Raja Yoga schools. These Kriyas affect the basic polarity of the body regulating the electrical flow in the nervous system and the ionisation of cellular energy. In Yoga it is taught that by the use of these Pranayama Kriyas and Prakriyas, deep relaxation can be produced, after which the higher Kriyas of the Laya Yoga and the Kundalini arousing Kriyas can be safely taught to qualified students.

Anu-Loma-Viloma Kriya 1

Anu Loma vilona kriya 1

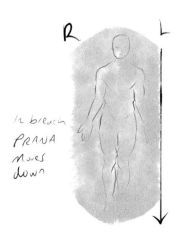

R   L

In breath
PRANA
moves
down

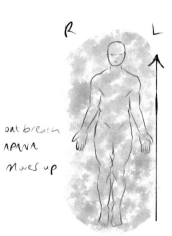

R   L

out breath
APANA
moves up

43

Technique: Lie down in the supine position, Shava Asana, the Corpse Posture. Have the head facing to the north to pick up the natural north-south flow of magnetic current. Begin deep rhythmic, Savitri Pranayama. Take in the breath for a slow eight count, hold in for a slow four count. Let out for a slow eight count, then hold out for a slow four count and repeat over and over again.

When you have mastery over the rhythmic Breath imagine that a warm golden Prana is flowing from above your head out the feet on the incoming breath. This Pranic flow is allowed to completely move beyond the feet. On the out-going breath, feel a cool silvery Apanic flow enter the feet and flow back through the body and out the top of the head. Continue this Pranic/Apanic flow until deep relaxation ensues, This should take six to ten minutes. A longer time may be used.

Anu-Loma-Viloma Kriya 2

Anu loma - viloma   kriya PART 2

R

L

In breath
PRANA

Out breath
APANA

Another form of polarity Kriya can be done by splitting apart the two flows so that the Apanic flow is felt to move downwards only on the left side of the body through Ida Nadi while the Pranic flow moves up on the right side of the body through Pingala Nadi. This Kriya is done over and over again until deep, conscious relaxation is produced.

Often the Guru will give a series of Nadas, Bijas or Mantras to "imagine" while doing the two Kriyas above. The beginner should imagine the Pranava "OM", being wafted in both directions with the breath through the body until given a more appropriate" Mantra. Such Mantras consist of the sound "Hang" on the out breath, and "Sah" on the in breath.

Other sounds popularly given are the sound "Ah", on the out breath and "Ee" on the in breath. In some Yoga systems the vowels of "Ah", "AAh", "I", "Ee", "U", "Oo". "Eh", "Ai", "Oh" "Au", "Huh" and "Mm" are circulated around the nervous system while doing similar Kriyas and Prakriyas. Using vowel sounds is incorrectly called Kriya Yoga and rightfully belongs in the Jnana Yoga system. Bijas and Mantras are used in the Laya Yoga Kriiyas as well as elaborate visualisation while doing appropriate Pranayamas, but such techniques can only be taught personally by a qualified Guru.

Cosmic Polarity

We are alive because of a harmonious interaction between our planet earth, its satellite moon, the sun which cores this part of our solar system, and our galactic and Cosmic source. If any single part of the Cosmic Harmony is disturbed, we are influenced; indeed, we may suffer greatly and perish. We all are aware of the effect of the moon on the water tides of this planet and the heave of the earth crust during the ebb and flow of a lunar cycle.

We observe the effect of solar rays flung into our ionosphere from our sun and the effects of sun spots on the penetration of solar rays into our atmosphere ... the increased danger of ultra-violet rays burning the skin and the effects of sun spots on our ability to concentrate and meditate. Bypassing comets are seen to affect us emotionally and mentally as they way-fare through celestial space. Whatever their effect, we are affected because we are a part of the whole Universe! "As above as below".

Though our earth spins madly on in time and space, we are blissfully unaware of its daily complete circuit on its polar axis. Yet, if our planet were to "slow down", we would be the victim of a slowing centrifugal force, affecting immediately the fluids of our body and especially our blood. If the speed of our planet were to increase, we would suffer a resultant centripetal aggravation creating a whole range of new physical and mental disorders.

Good old Mother Earth remains a safe and sure Mother for us, while the polarity of the planet remains as it is. The slightest shift of our planets molten core would change the magnetic poles and life as we know it on Earth would have to change drastically. Earth scientists claim that has happened many hundreds of times over the millions of years of the life of planet Earth.

This accounts for the strange fact that we find tropical jungles as coal seams thousands of metres beneath the earth and the petroleum products which we bring up from the bowels of the earth are the remnants of long- gone insects and swamp plants. We find sea shells thousands of metres up the new mountains of the earth like the Himalayas, the Andes and the Rocky Mountains. The mind is awed by past earth changes… when the earth lost its polarity briefly. Imagine what would happen to us if we lost our own personal polarity?

Every cell in the human body has a duplicate polarity to the planet Earth. Just as our mother planet is bombarded by Cosmic Neutrinos, so also our body is constantly penetrated by these fast moving energy particles. Perhaps Science will soon decide that these energy particles are the Prana we talk of in Yoga at its Cosmic level. The Prana associated with the breath we breathe is stimulated within our atmosphere by the bombardment of Cosmic Prana from the very core of the Cosmos. This Prana maintains the polarity of every cell in our body if we are good, deep breathers.

The electrical potential of our cells is vitally maintained by the anion-cation exchange of energy. Electrolytic balance of each cell is the result of this Prana-Breath-Cellular interaction. Electrolytic balance is maintained whether we are standing, sitting, kneeling squatting, lying face prone or supine on the back if we are healthy, emotionally well balanced and good deep breathers. For those who are morose, destructive of thought, negative of emotions, hypochondriacal, and shallow breathers, the natural polarity suffers through entropy. Cellular polarity is lost, and the cell dies. Whole organs may be affected and ultimately the complete body.

We suffer much by default, not knowing that the great secret of life is in the breath. Yogis have discovered this vital knowledge and have passed it on to their followers. Hence, in Yoga, the directives to eschew bad habits and debilitating vices, to leave off harmful foods and those which distort polarity, leaving us depolarised. Yoga as Union could be defined as "right polarity". "Nara : Psychic Disassociation", is term for imbalanced polarity which Swamiji mentions "I think that you will find the answer for most perplexing problems about emotional imbalance, mental disorders and those seemingly hard-to-cure physical disorders, which in Yoga we describe as "non-disease diseases" in the concept of Nara.

Alu-Loma-Viloma Prakriyas

If you get confused with all the terms used in Yoga for its various Kriyas and Prakriyas, then you are to be excused. There are so many terms to remember, and later recall. This is the proof that Yoga is a great science, and you must be prepared to learn its gigantic vocabulary, so that you can understand Its techniques and processes. Such understanding is typified by the Yoga Prakriya called Alu-Loma-Viloma, a part of the Polarity Kriya series.

The term "Alu" used for this Prakriya Is a shortened form of "Alaya, an abode or dwelling place, a receptacle or vessel suggested as the vital body, the psychic body which is also called Pranamaya Kosha. The word "Aalu" also means a raft or a kind of boat made up of floats and alludes to the states of the body after doing this Prakriya. The technique is also referred to as Aaluchana Kriya, a Kriya used to "rend, apart' or "tear apart" old Karmic holds of the "lower nature". My students often jokingly remind me that "Alu" also means a "potato" or "tuber root".

Whatever the term, it will become extraordinarily clear as you undertake the technique. There is a resemblance between this Prakriya and the Anu-Loma Vitoma Kriya. While doing parts of this technique, one can use the sound of AUM, HANG and SAH or the sound of AH or EE. Using these Bijas is often taken to be a part of the Kundalini arousing Layas Yoga techniques which are taught only to the most advanced students, and only in the presence of a highly qualified Guru.

The purpose of this Alu - Loma -Viloma Prakriya is to get one centred into the channels associated with the energy flow in the spinal area. These practices are often accompanied by Pranayama techniques like Ujjayi and Surya Bhedana. This Kriya will ensure that the other practices are fruitful, but has an additional deep relaxation effect upon those who constantly use this technique. It has much to be recommended as a relaxation technique after a lengthy session of Pranayama or at the end of a good Hatha Yoga workout to reinforce the benefits of the physical activity.

There are two great fluxes of Prana energy at play through the human body. One Is associated with the incoming breath, and referred to as Prana. The second is associated with the discharge of the breath, and is called Apana. These terms at this particular point are rather arbitrarily used, as there are actually twelve terms associated with Prana. Five of these are said to be major Pranas, called the Pancha Prana Vayus. Another five, the Upa-Prana Vayus, are called the Minor Vital Airs while two others are referred to as Akasha Vayu and Chitta Vayu.

Alu-Loma-Viloma Prakriya 1

The Alu-Loma Viloma Prakriya can be done as three distinct Kriyas or consecutively, one after the other, as a Prakriya. In Part I, lie down with the head to the north to take advantage of the natural north-south polarity of our planet earth. Do a few rounds of polarity breath Anu-Loma-Viloma. The breathing should be in the style of Savitri Pranayama, an 8:4:8:4 ratio.

After a few rounds of Polarity Breath, imagine that you are lying in the giant oval of energy which extends 15cms (six inches) above the head and 15cms (six inches) below the feet, and can be divided completely into two halves, one on the right side of the body, and one on the left side of the body. On an out-going breath, let the Apanic flow move down the left side of the body from head to feet. Hold a point below the feet for the short count. Now draw in the breath and feel the rising Pranic flow on the right side of the oval to the top of the head. Continue this "ovaling" of energy for a minimum of nine complete rounds of the breath. Many more rounds of breath can be used if one has the time. A marvellous sense of "psychic protection" will be felt by doing this Kriya, and perhaps this is the origin of placing a mystic circle of energy right around one's body to ward off the negative thoughts of others, and the effects of psychic accidents.

Part 1

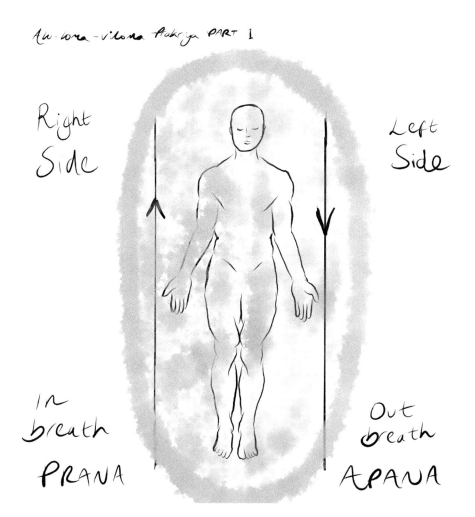

Anu-loma-viloma Prakriya PART 1

Right Side

Left Side

In breath PRANA

Out breath APANA

Part 2

Alu-Loma-Viloma Pakriya PART 2   (Smaller ovaling)

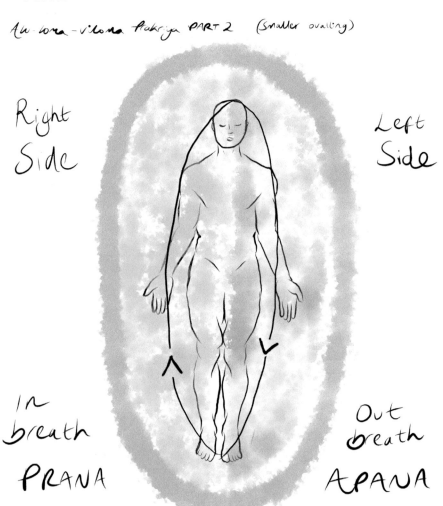

Right Side

Left Side

In breath
PRANA

Out breath
APANA

Imagine the oval somewhat restricted to take in an area from the top of the head to the feet and continue the same Apanic flow on the out breath down the left side of the oval, while the Pranic flow is drawn up the right side of the oval. Continue this smaller "ovaling" of the breath for a minimum of nine rounds, or the same number of rounds, that you have done in Part I of Alu-Loma-Viloma

Prakriya. This part of the Kriya will give you the sense of being self-contained and self-reliant while also producing a marvellous sense of relaxation and well-being.

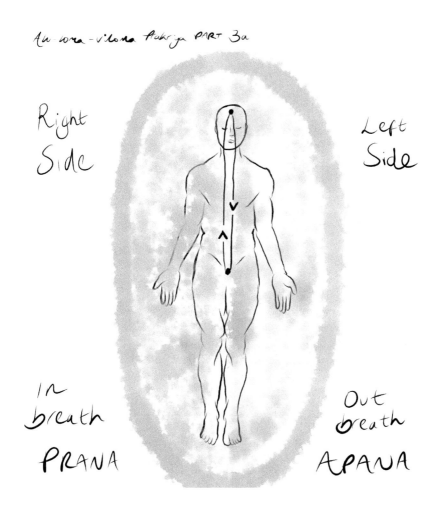

Anu-oma-viloma Prakriya PART 3a

Right Side

Left Side

In breath

PRANA

Out breath

APANA

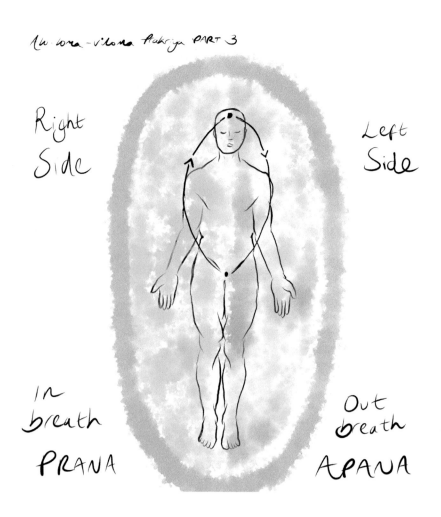

Right Side

Left Side

In breath

PRANA

Out breath

APANA

Part 3

Restrict the oval movement of the Prana/ Apana to a point within the centre of the brain and the base of the spine. Move the Apanic flow downwards on the outgoing breath and the Pranic flow upwards on the in breath. The breathing is still Rhythmic Breath, although there may be a desire to omit the held in and the held out part of the breath. If this arises spontaneously, then the urge may be safely followed.

After about nine rounds of this "ovaling" breath, the energy flow may be further restricted so that it is moving like a narrow loop up Pingala Nadi, the right peripheral channel of the spine and down Ida Nadi, the left peripheral channel of the spine. Continue the entire Prakriya until the deepest sense of relaxation ensues.

This part of the Kriya produces the deepest sense of positive relaxation. In a sense it may also be the "lull before the storm" if one were to proceed on into Kundalini-arousing Laya Yoga Kriyas, because the next step would be to follow a similar procedure while in a sitting posture, and then consciously doing a Pranayama like Surya Bhedana the Sun-energy splitting Pranayama.

Part 4

Alu-Loma-Viloma Prakriya Part 4

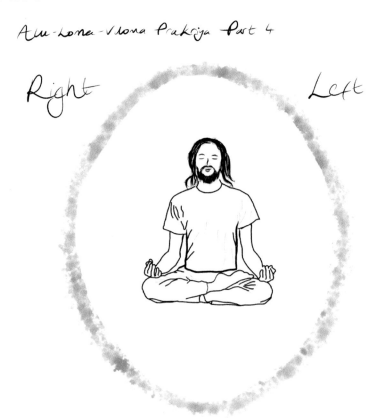

Right   Left

It is possible to do Alu-Loma Viloma Prakriya while sitting. It is best to learn this Kriya while lying with the head to the North in Shava Asana . This will ensure that your Spine is straight until you learn to sit Yogically erect for sitting postures, Kriyas and Prakriyas, in a Yogic position are fruitless practices. The best way to get a good Yoga posture is to be aware of your everyday movement while walking, sitting, resting and relaxing. One can do a world of good to an otherwise un-yogic spine by watchful awareness. Doing a little Yoga once in a while may not straighten the spine and especially if Asanas are done without awareness.

When that awareness of good posture comes, sit in Sukha Asana, Siddha Asana, Ardha Padma Asana, or Padma Asana, facing to the North.

Remove as many sight and sound distractions as humanly possible, then, imagine a giant oval of energy which extends both below the sitting position and above the top of the head. For the first few rounds, simply imagine a giant oval of energy with its ecliptic both above and below the body. Make sure that the energy visualised encompasses the body, and the visualisation is not "on top of the body".

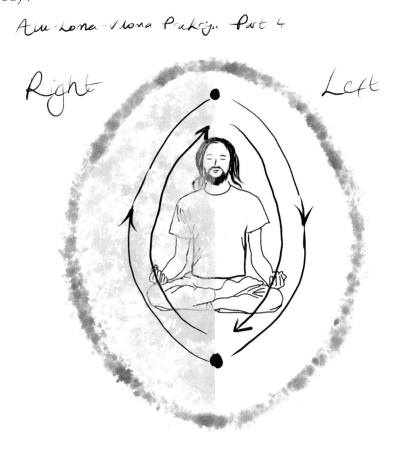

Now, feel positive warm Pranic flow on the right side of the oval, moving from the negative base ecliptic up the right side of the oval to the positive point of the ecliptic above the head. Start with an oval that is about 15cms. (6 inches) above and below the body. Slowly extend this oval in size until it is 60cms. (two feet) below the sitting position and as much as a full metre (3 feet) above the head. It helps to be sitting on solid ground, sand, or rock if possible for this Kriya. It may not have the most positive effects if you are doing this on the tenth floor of a high—rise apartment as the "ground" to which one should be "grounded" is not there.

Anu-Loma-Viloma Prakriya Part 4

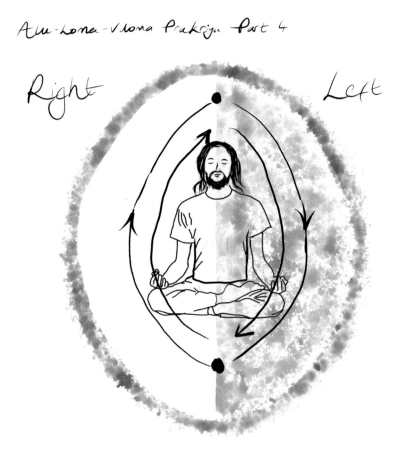

Right   Left

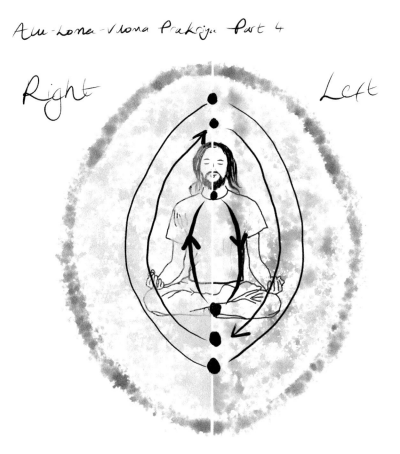

Further restrict and visualise the oval to just below the sitting body and just above the top of the head. Warm, golden Prana flows up the right side of the oval on the in breath, and cool silvery Apana flows down on the left side of the oval. if nine rounds of this Prakriya were done on the outer oval, then continue at least nine or more rounds on this second oval.

Now restrict the Prana-Apana to a point at the base of the spine and at the back of the throat palate. Repeat a minimum of nine rounds of the Pranic flow on the right side of the oval and the Apanic flow on the left side of the oval. In this more restricted track, a larger number of rounds may be done to heighten neurological polarity associated with Ida Nadi on the right side of the body, and Pingala Nadi on the left side of the body. This will increase the energy stored up in the Kanda (Conus Medularis) and allow for a uni-polar energy arousal.

Prana Vayus – Subtle Psychic Energy Currents

Swara Yoga explains that all our physical, mental, emotional and spiritual functions of body-mind are governed by Prana Vayus which are the positive and negative ions like electric or magnetic forces. These are various energy currents flowing through various Nadis or energy channels supporting particular areas of our body and mind. There are ten important Prana Vayus regulating and distributing vital energy throughout the body. Out of these, the five major Prana Vayus are Prana, Apana, Samana, Udana, and Vyana.

The Prana Vayu is situated in the thoracic region, absorbs incoming vital energy from air elements and creates upward movements of energy for heart, lungs and chest region. The Apana Vayu is opposite to Prana Vayu and causes energy to move downwards for the reproductive and excretory organs in the lower body. The two energy currents also play an important role in polarity in our body and energy.

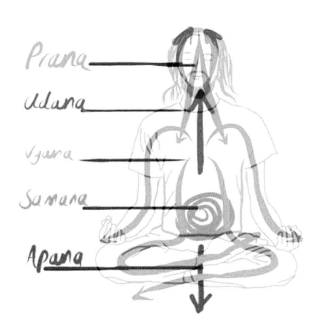

Samana is the third of these Vayus governing digestive functions, and resonates in abdominal areas. The Udana Vayu moves and vibrates in the throat and face areas and regulates swallowing and facial activities. Vyana Vayus circulates or flows throughout the whole body and hence becomes a connecting force. This regulates all physical movements by supplying food and nutrients throughout the whole body.

Out of the five Prana Vayus, Prana-Apana Vayus are most powerful and regulate and or influence all other three Prana Vayus. In Tantra and Upanishads, it is said that "when the two opposite energy currents Prana-Apana are united, all the other Prana Vayus naturally attain harmony".

Role of Balance of Positive-Negative ions for Health

The Yogis and followers of Tantra, Samkhya, and Swara Yoga explained that these positive-negative energies known as Prana-Apana, Loma-Viloma, Suriya-Chanra, Shakti-Shiva are charged in the atmosphere or the universe and body absorbs them and through our Chakra system revitalise the Dasha-Vayus or ten subtle energies, which are governing or sustaining psycho-physiological functions associated with fields of their operations.

Some modern research has been done where healthy and dynamic people were exposed to an environment with a high positive ion content and found this caused lethargy and drowsiness.

Some of them complained of headaches and respiratory issues. Longer exposure to excessive positive ions also produced euphoria and mental agitation. On the other hand, after exposure to a high concentration of negative ions, physical and mental capacities were revitalised and invigorated.

Swamiji Dr Gitananda Giriji mentions that over populated areas, with excess of machines, electric appliances, and all sorts of electro-magnetic frequencies have a huge negative impact on the balance of these positive and negative ions.

If the environment is depleted from these positive and negative ions or energies, you will easily find the plants and animal growth will be inhibited by the low ionisation. If we remove these particles completely from the air, food, water, etc it will become lifeless and poisonous. We need this polarity, and balance, as well as an abundance of positive-negative ions or energy in the atmosphere to be healthy or even to live.

Our ecologists are showing us that the modern pollution of our technology, internet, wifi, television and radio frequencies are destroying this balance of negative and positive ions. This is unnaturally affecting our health, and wellbeing. You will be surprised to find that these days there are machines available to buy to enhance ionisation in your home or workplace for survival. This imbalanced ionisation also impacts our Dasa-Vayu or ten-subtle energy currents in our body. People living in rural areas can easily experience this every time they go to stay in big cities due to excess of electro-magnetic pollution and depletion of ionisation, they may suffer with lack of good sleep, headaches, lethargy, indigestion etc.

However it may not be easy for us as an individuals to change all this, but by learning Swara Yoga and applying the practices, pranayama, kriyas and prakriyas we can easily manipulate our energy systems and enhance our health and wellbeing. Our modern science is working tirelessly on exploring our macro-cosmos, which is priceless. Swara Yoga explores our micro-cosmos and its relation with macro-cosmos and teaches us how to utilise these energy principles in relation to finding harmony or balance in our inner environment. We can live in total harmony by adhering to laws of nature and intoning with biorhythms.

Our Nostrils: A Subtle Energy Detector

We all are aware and know it very well that our life and biological survival is dependent on breathing. We are living beings as long as we are breathing, the moment we stop breathing, our life also stops. The Hatha Yoga Pradipika mentions in the second chapter that, "as long as breathing continues, life exists, when breath departs, soul or life also departs, therefor regulate the breath." If we start thing, how do I regulate my breath or how do I manipulate it? Our nostrils become the easiest points to begin. It is easy to be aware or notice the pattern of breathing in our nostrils as well as by closing them and opening them in various patterns we can easily change the breathing pattern. For this reason Swara Yoga begins with examining the flow of air in the nose and pattern of nostril breathing.

Our nasal cavity is uniquely designed for various purposes. This allows a safe entry and exit of air for the life process, it also has a soft lining and hair stricture to stop all the unsafe particles entering the air passage. This cavity also detects the Suriya-Chandra or Pranic energy ionisation.

This nasal cavity is made of thin, perforated bone known as cribriform plate of the ethmoid bone. Within these perforations there are the minute filaments of the olfactory nerve. These nerves send all the information to the brain regarding constituents, and the quality of the air we breathing in. When Pranic charged ions come in contact with these nerve endings and filaments, the brain and main nervous system automatically gets stimulated and become energised. These charging electric impulses travel to the limbic system of the brain, where perception is transformed into experience. So, in this way our breathing directly affects our mental and emotional responses to life situations and events, and vice-versa the arousal of different mental and emotional activities can be easily reflected in the breath. If we breath through the mouth, our Prana and breath moves straight down in trachea or windpipe without stimulating our brain and nervous system. Hence activation and stimulation of our nervous system and brain has certain dependence on our nasal breathing.

Further to extend this, the nerves in our right nostril are connected with the left brain and the nerves in our left nostril are connected with the right brain. Hence when we breathing predominantly through right nostrils, our left brain is predominantly stimulated or charged, while when we breathing through the left nostril, our right brain is predominantly stimulated or charged. This means that activation of our intellectual, artistic, creative, maths, and other skills also have a direct connection with our breathing patterns. According to Swara Yoga, "knowing your Swaras are like knowing the waves and how to ride them to become a great surfer".

Absorption of Ions or Pranic Force in Our Body

Once the Vayu or air enters the nasal cavity, it activates all the nasal nerves and then enters the windpipe and moves into both our lungs. In our lungs in alveoli cells, the exchange of gases -oxygen and carbon dioxide occurs as part of our breathing and the same also happens at cellular level. In this process to fully utilise the Prana energy in our body a certain chemical and energetic breakdown or release has to take place. It is like refining the crude fuels into refined petrol or diesel for our cars. This releases an abundance of

Pranic vital force and hence Yogis describe slower and rhythmic breathing to fully utilise this potential energy from each breath to revitalise our body, mind and soul.

Negative ions, known as Shakti are the body energisers as they work as the catalysts for the ionisation and oxygenation of the blood as well as at cellular level to enhance metabolic activities and abundance of energy release. This generates heat and energy for our life process. This energy travels via our blood stream to facilitate digestion for further breakdown of food to release and absorb all the nutrients our bodies need for healthy functioning. If there is an excess of positive ions, it retards our metabolic activities and this energy release process. This results in poor digestion, lack of energy, improper oxygenation and ionisation. This energy distribution shows us the flow of Prana Vayus and their correlation with certain functions in our body affected by positive and negative ions or Ida and Pingala Swaras.

The Cosmic Exchange and Balance

During inhalation we receive or take in the energies of the universe in their seed potential form with all the cosmic codes of wisdom and existence and with exhalation we are sending all the information of our individual environment back to the universe or cosmos. Here the shakti or potential energy transforms into life forces during inhalation then all the residues and individual energies send back to the universe to have the perfect balance between our internal and external environment. It can be simply seen as a perfect communication between micro and macro-cosmos during breathing.

In Tantra inhalation or Puraka is known as Shakti and exhalation of Rechaka is known as Shiva. In Pranayama Yoga, we also learn to retain or hold the breath in and out. Inner retention of breath is known as Antar Kumbhaka and external retention of breath is known as Bahir Kumbhaka. Tantra explains that state of Kumbhaka and allows the Shakti and Shiva to unite and resonate, pulsate or dance together.

Swara Yoga and Modern Energy Principle

Modern science as well as Ancient wisdom principles detail that nature's creation and existence is essentially due to transmission, transmutation, transformation and evolution of potential energy and consciousness. In Samkhya it is said the whole universe is created from Prana – the subtle cosmic force, Akasha – ethereal space, Purusha -the consciousness and Prakriti -primordial nature qualities or wisdom. This universal evolution or progression is based on effortless dynamic transformation. Our body, mind and life are also part of this effortless natural transformation and subject to all the changes.

Our modern scientists have found so many ways to control and manipulate many aspects of natural forces as well as producing forces like electricity, all these appliances, huge turbines, machines, radio waves, etc. With modern technology we can produce energy to power our cities, and transmit messages not only across the earth but even beyond. We can communicate or transmit information to various planets.

The Yogic journey obviously is the opposite to this modern science approach. Yogic and Rishis found that we can experience the universe and all these forces by going inward and connecting our individual body, breath, prana, mind and consciousness. Swara Yoga teaches us how to know, refine, control or manipulate these divine forces in our body to boost our health, immunity and accelerate spiritual evolutionary journey.

We can see this energy transmutation on a large scale in our wind turbines and hydro-power stations. Here the power of wind or water flow is used to rotate the turbines encompassed in a strong magnetic field, producing electric power. This power is transformed or transported via the cables and again used to power lights, all devices and appliances where this electric energy is changed into kinetic energy in so many appliances. The energy production, transmutation and transportation is quite similar to the same principles.

The Yogis describe various Pranic fields, Prana Vayus, Chakras, Nadis and how respiration generates energy and transforms in various forms, flows through Nadis, resonates through Chakras and flows in various physical, mental, pranic and spiritual areas. This energy is mainly produced, transformed and stored in the main plexuses along the spinal column known as Chakras in Yoga.

Once these electric currents are produced or stored, they can only be transferred or transported in specific voltages via suitable cables. In our body, channels or energy wires are known as Nadis and turbines or dynamos are known as Chakras. This cosmic Prana or vital energy is produced or transformed in our Chakras and then released into Prana Nadis in the form of Prana Vayus. These energies have three qualities - positive, negative or neutral. The Prana Vayus Nadis also take on characteristics and qualities of the particular energy and their qualities flowing through them.

Nadis

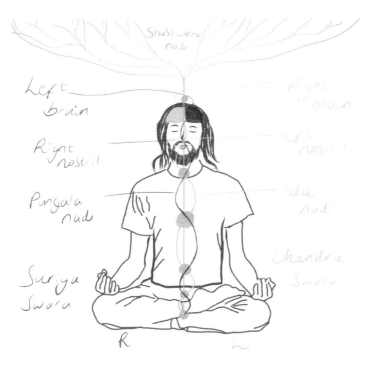

The Varaha-Upanishad (v.54-5) mentions that: "Nadis are infused in the body from the soles of the feet to the crown of the head, carrying Prana, the breath of life, in which abides the Atman, and the source of Shakti, the living or creating force of all the worlds." These Nadis have their seat of existence in our Pranamaya Kosha and are known as meeting points with our physical and mental bodies.

Hatha Yoga Pradipika and Goraksha Samhita mentions 72,000 Nadis while Shiva Samhita mentions a total of 350,000 Nadis emerging from the Navel. These Nadis are dscribed as a thin thread or tubes connecting with lotus stems of Chakras hanging down and supported by the spinal column. The Anatomy of the nervous system described by modern medical science shows the clear correlation with the description of Nadis. Here Chakras can be related with the nerve plexus. Out of these Nadis fourteen are major or important Nadis. Of these, three Nadis known as Ida, Pingala and Sushumna are the most important.

In Recent Yoga work by many scholarly yoga masters, the network of the Nadis has been literally interpreted as being identical with the nervous system. But the Chandogya and Brihadaranyaka Upanishads clearly explain that the Nadis are entirely subtle in nature and they don't have their existence in the physical body. The word 'Nadi' comes from the Sanskrit root 'nad', which refers to the resonating vibrations in a hollow tube.

If one considers roots as Nadis in a plant pot, then earth can be considered as our body. We can clearly see how earth and roots are supporting each other and infused together. They both are in mutual transformation for plant or life to blossom, but still they are completely separate. Similarly our Pranic Nadis and physical body are infused or interlinked but still are separate in existence. Teleportation and astral travel can be understood under this phenomenon easily and scientifically.

This Yogic idea of Pranic Nadi network is unique but in recent years some scientists are investigating the electromagnetic currents of plants, animals, various organs in our body and nervous system. Dr.

R. Becker of New York, in his 5 year study, measured and analysed the electrical emissions from the cells lining the exterior walls of the peripheral nerves. He found that a constant current is always flowing, even though the nerves themselves only react when they are stimulated, at which point this energy current also changes in power and frequency. These energy currents are much stronger along the nervous system.

The micro-electric impulses are travelling along or within the nervous system, carrying the messages from brain to cells and vice-versa. This transmission of energy flow can be seen as equivalent to Pranic flow in Nadis. Neuroscience can measure the alpha, beta and gama energy waves of our brain in various states of our body, mind and emotions. Our Chandra and Suriya Swaras can be interlinked with our sympathetic and parasympathetic nervous system. But we can physically explore and study nervous system, while the Swaras or Nadis are experiential through Yoga Sadhana.

The Shiva Swarodaya also mentions that out of these thousands of Nadis, ten are most significant because they are the connections to the 'doorways' leading in and out of the body. Seven of these Nadis have lesser influence.

These seven are:
1. Gandhari, connecting to the left eye
2. Hastijihva, connecting to the right eye
3. Pusha, connecting to the right ear
4. Yashaswini, connecting to the left ear
5. Alambusha, connecting to the mouth
6. Kuhu, connecting to the reproductive organs
7. Shankhini, connecting to the rectum.

The three most important Nadis are Ida, Pingala and Sushumna, which we may correspond with the parasympathetic, sympathetic and cerebrospinal nervous systems. These channels have great significance because they are the conductors of the negative, positive and neutral energies.

Ida is the left Nostril or Chandra Swara. Ida is white, silver, feminine, cooling, and represents the Chandra or moon. This is associated with the river Ganga (Ganges). Ida is originating in Mooladhara, and merges or ends in the left nostril.

Pingala is the right Nostril or Suriya Swara. Pingala is red, masculine, warming, and represents the Suriya or sun. PIngala is associated with the river Yamuna. Pingala originates in Mooladhara, and merges or ends in the right nostril.

Sushumna is the central or balanced channel, when breath flows equally through both nostrils. This is associated with the river Saraswati. Within the Sushumna nadi there are three more subtle Nadis: Vajra, Chitrini and Brahma Nadi. Kundalini flows upwards through the Sushumna from Mooladhara to Sasashrara Chakra.

The kanda (energy store) in Mooladhara Chakra is the origin place of the three main nadis and is known as Yukta Triveni (Yukta: "combined", Tri: "three", Veni: "streams"). In Mooladhara, Shakti, the latent potential un-manifested Kundalini, is symbolised by a serpent coiled into three and a half circles around the central axis Svayambhu-Linga at the base of the spine. The serpent lies blocking the entrance to Sushumna, the central channel.

Sushumna Swara or Channel in context to its full potential remains closed at its lower end as long as the Kundalini is not awakened. This is why kundalini awakening or Kundalini Yoga is one of the important classical Yoga Sadhana paths.

Kundalini Yoga provides tools for enhancing Prana vibrations or energy and guide its flow through Ida and Pingala Swaras or Nadis into the Mooladhara Chakra and then allows the awakened energy to flow upward through the central channel known as Sushumna Nadi. Swara Yoga describes that the balance of Nadis can be achieved by controlled switching between Nadis or Swaras. This will gradually unify the Shakti and Shiva or Chandra and Suriya Nadis which will lead onto the awakening of Kundalini. Once awakened this energy will flow upward energising each of Chakra. Once the Crown Chakra opens, Sadhaka experiences Sat-Chit-Ananda, a state of divine bliss.

From Mooladhara chakra, Ida and Pingala Nadis are moving upward in a criss-crossing way and alternating from the right to left side and left to right side at each chakra until they merge in Ajna chakra where they meet again with Sushumna.

In Ajna chakra the union or merging of the three main nadis is known as Mukta Triveni (Mukta: "liberated", Tri: "three", Veni: "streams") Ida, Chandra or the Negative Energy.

The Ida Nadi Chandra or negative charge

The Swara Yoga scriptures explain that negative ions, or energy, flows through the Ida Nadi as the flow of Chitta the mental energy. Because the lunar energy passes along this channel, it is also known as Chandra Nadi. Ida plays a role in cooling and quietening the processes of the body and functions correspond with the parasympathetic nervous system.

The Ida Nadi governs the left side of the body. This Nadi originates at the left side of the sacro-coccygeal plexus and terminates at the root of the left nostril. From the origin point at Mooladhara Chakra in the base of the spine, Ida Nadi spirals upwards, intersecting the vertebral column in the four main plexuses, or chakras. Stimulation of Ida Nadi enriches all these Chakras with Negative ions.

The Ida Nadi and the parasympathetic system show a significant relationship as they both have a calming influence on the body and the mind. This energy allows the energy to flow inward and conserve energy for the activation of the visceral organs, promoting secretions of digestive enzymes in the digestive tract, increasing peristalsis and emptying the bladder. This further relaxes the heart, breathing, and reduces muscle stress.

As the stress levels are reduced, our key organs relax, this further relaxes our mind and nervous system. So it improves mental focus and awareness. When we become aware, the nervous system is relaxed, clarity of thought and choices improve naturally. Even our taste, smell, desires, and thoughts naturally seek out healthier ones. This enhances of our mental creativity, psychic abilities, spiritual virtues and higher thoughts.

It is interesting to also see scientifically when the Ida Nadi and or Parasympathetic Nervous System is active, our pupils are constricted and the eye lenses are adjusted to bring the objects at close range in focus, which is decreasing external input to the visual cortex of our brain. Chandra or Ida Swara can be activated to relax our heart, breathing, nervous system, muscles, and activate our digestive functions. Also, before relaxation and concentration practice activation of this Chandra energy will help us to focus bringing a more introverted energy.

The Pingala, Surya or Positive Charge

The Pingala, or Surya is the counterpart of the Ida Nadi or energy channel. It is the transmitter and channel of the Prana, or positive energy, from, the Sun or Surya. The Pingala Nadi originates on the opposite of the Ida Nadi on the right side of the sacro-coccygeal plexus and merges or terminates at the root of the right nostril. The Pingala Nadi dominates the right side of our body. Likewise the Ida Nadi, Pingala Nadi also spirals upward along the vertebral column, intersecting the Ida and Sushumna Nadi at the four main Chakras or energy plexuses. This positive aspect Prana flowing through this Nadi, recharges all our Chakras with positive energy.

The Pingala Nadi correlates all its functions with our sympathetic nervous system by activating extrovert vital energy. This also leads our mind, nervous system and ego to feel energised and active. This is similar with the release of the adrenaline hormone in our bloodstream when the sympathetic nervous system is dominating. This accelerates heartbeat, blood pressure, further causing constriction of blood vessels in the skin and digestive tract. This diverts blood in superficial muscles and organs of action, and slows down peristalsis movement and digestion activities. Eye pupils are dilated, which allows a broader range of vision and increased fields of sensory input to our brain. Our awareness is externalised. To consciously activate, control or change these functions and energy, a Yogic needs to learn and master how to manipulate this energy in Pingala Nadi or Swara.

Transformation of The Ida and Pingala

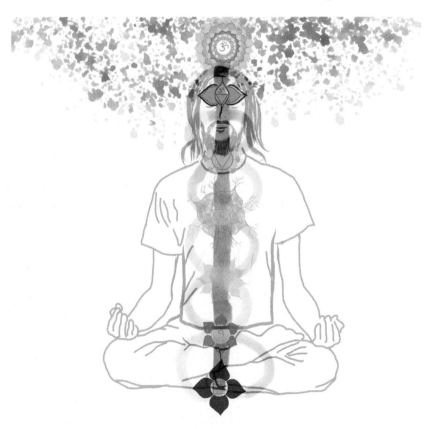

Understanding the idea of the Ida and Pingala; Loma-Viloma; Shiva Shakti divides our body in two parts - right and left, positive and negative or sun and moon. As these energies are meeting and criss-crossing in the middle and creating another energy field, which is neutral in nature. This is the field or energy channel of the Sushumna Nadi. Sushumna Nadi travels upward through the centre of our vertebral column, corresponding with the functions of the central or cerebrospinal nervous system.

Sushumna Nadi also originates at the mid point of the sacra-coccygeal plexus along with the Ida at the left and the Pingala at the right. Sushumna Nadi follows a straight path upward, piercing all the main Chakras or energy plexuses. This is really the energy channel which is in the interest of every Yoga Sadhaka seeking spiritual experiences. This Nadi is dormant in everyone, obviously there is very little flow of energy in this channel for our basic spiritual needs. The Hatha Yoga Pradipika in chapter 2 mentions that, "Sushumna Nadi remains dormant due to the impurities of the Nadis". Once the Sushumna Nadi opens, the two opposite energies of Ida and Pingala flows through this middle channel and Sushumna and balanced energy becomes the life governing principle.

While our Sushumna Nadi is dormant, all the other Nadis, energies and life governing principles are under the influence of the positive-negative energy duality of the Ida and Pingala Nadi. We mostly live under the influence of the Ida or Pingala Nadi depending on the flow of breath through the left or right nostril. When the breath flows equally through both the nostrils, these positive and negative energies find the perfect balance and energy flows in freely through the Sushumna as the Kundalini awakens. This free us from duality and lead us to Oneness, Union, Harmony and self-realisation.

Here is the table or various symbolic representations and relatedness of these subtle life energies.

Ida Nadi	Pingala Nadi	Sushumna Nadi
Negative ions	Positive ions	Neutral ions
Feminine energy	Masculine energy	Neutral energy
Viloma	Loma	Soma
Chandra	Surya	Balance
Lunar	Solar	Fire
Yin	Yang	Tao
Night	Day	Dusk, and Dawn
Shakti	Shiva	Union of Shiva-Shakti
Space	Time	Matter
Consciousness	Activity	Bliss
Cold	Hot	Soothing
Mind field	Vital field	Super-conscious field
Chitta	Prana	Kundalini
Desire	Action	Wisdom
Subconscious Field	Conscious field	Unconscious and Super-conscious field
Passive	Active	Centred
Parasympathetic	Sympathetic	Cerebrospinal
Yamuna river	Ganga river	Saraswati river
Creative force	Dissolution force	Liberating force
White or Silver	Red or Golden	Black
Brahma	Vishnu	Shiva or Rudra
Akaar	Ukaar	Makaar

Symbolic Representation of the Trinity Of Nadis or Swaras

According to quantum science, all matter are evolutes of the subtlest form of energy known as quanta. This energy takes many forms and goes through transformation and manifestation, evolution and involution, but still remains preserved. This nature enables creation to sustain it as well as dissolve it back to the source or energy. These energies are further broken down or explained as protons, neutrons and electrons similar to the Ida, Pingala and Sushumna energies.

Sushumna or the central channel is the subtlest of the three Nadis and also contains all the three primordial qualities known as Tamas, Rajas and Sattva. When the energy flows in harmony, it refines the subtle qualities and the Sadhakas gradually progress into Sattva as full awakening, Sadhakas attains freedom from the Tri-Gunas, and Samaskaras.

The external structure of Sushumna Nadi is related to the quality of Tamas, as it is inert. Within this we have the Vajra Nadi related with the Tamas. Innermost lies the Chittra Nadi related to the Sattva. The furthest and deepest of this lies the subtlest Nadi known as Brahma Nadi. When the conscious energy flows through the Brahma Nadi, it leads the Sadhaka to absolute realisation of the supreme consciousness known as Brahman.

The true aim of any form of Yoga is to awaken the Sushumna Nadi and direct the flow of the Prana in Sushumna Nadi to activate and recharge all the layers, through the union of the Ida and Pingala energy. Here Sadhaka becomes free from the dualistic nature of two opposite life forces and attains absolute harmony or balance known as Samattva and Samadhi.

Chakras

Chakra, meaning "wheel" or "circle", are psychic energy centres. These exist along the axis of the spine or three major Nadis in our Pranamaya Kosha. These Chakras hold conscious Prana potentials. These Wheels are represented in the form of lotuses. The Chakras don't have physical or material existence in our physical body or Annamaya Kosha. Chakras can be known as the little dynamos transforming universal Pranic forces into Prana Vayus governing our psycho-physio-spiritual activities. In this way we can visualise Chakras as a meeting point or junction between Pranamaya (subtle energy body) and Annamaya (food or physical body) and Manomaya (Mind body).

Just to remember that Chakras exist in Pranamaya Kosha. Also they are not stuck against our spine at the back as we might see them most publications. These Chakras are lotuses at each point from centre meeting point of Ida, Pingala and Sushumna Nadi and lotus like a disc spinning around the spinal axis.

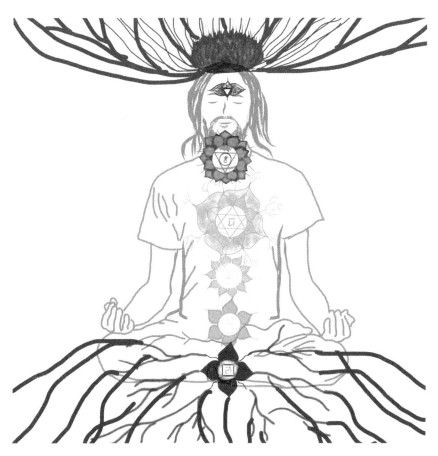

In Tantra there is mention of various numbers of Chakras. The Seven Chakra system is generally known by most Yoga Sadhakas. Swamiji Dr Gitananda Giriji Mentions that there are 12 Chakras. Seven Chakras exist along our spine from Mooladhara to Sahashrara and the other 5 Chakras exist beyond our crown at the top in the sphere. This Chakras are higher or cosmic Chakras.

When kundalini is awakened at Mooladhara, it uncoils and begins to flow upwards like a fiery serpent, awakening or recharging each Chakra as it ascends, until the Shakti merges with Shiva in Sahashrara Chakra.

Each Chakra represents various levels of consciousness, regulating various physical, mental, emotional and spiritual functions. These energies are not positive or negative in the sense of quality and hence Yamas and Niyamas or ethical and moral values are to be mastered before we begin the spiritual journey of Kundalini awakening.

Seven Chakras

In our pranic body we have seven chakras. These are junction points where our major naris – Ida, Pingala, and Sushumna are meeting or criss-crossing each other. If you imagine shapes of eight on top of each others, that is how it will look with a straight line through the middle of them.

The first chakra is located at the base of the spine and is known as the Mooladhara (the root or foundation) Chakra. This is the chakra where kundalini rests coiled up in the form of a serpent. Our seventh chakra is known as the Sahashrara (thousand petals) chakra and it is based at the top of our head or crown. All the Yogis aim to open these two chakras to attain self-realisation or Samadhi.

The other five chakras define our personality and who we truly are. They also govern various psych-physiological functions in our body and hence blockages or imbalance of any of these chakras result into physical or mental health problems associated to those chakras, hence the balance of these chakras is key to a balanced health and well being.

Our second chakra is known as the Swadhisthana (self-dwelling place) chakra. This is based around our pelvic area and it is associated with the reproductive organs and kidneys. This chakra is naturally active or awakened in most human beings as part of the natural process to reproduce life and to sustain the life processes. The energy from this chakra flows and expresses itself through sensual or sexual pleasures in a gross form. While in subtle form it expresses or fulfils life through arts and creativity.

Our third chakra is known as the Manipura (jewel city) Chakra. This chakra is associated with the solar plexus, stomach, liver, pancreas and upper digestive system. This is the centre of the fire element and provides us with the necessary life forces to fulfil our karma and dharma. When this chakra is fully open we feel strong, brave and fearless while, if it is blocked, we are fearful, anxious and worried.

Our forth chakra is the Anahata (unstruck) chakra. It is associated with heart and lungs. This chakra gives us force to give and receive unconditional joy, love and happiness. When this chakra, is blocked, we feel a lack of faith or trust in ourselves or others and tend to be more self-centred. While, when it is open fully, we feel positive, confident, caring and nurturing towards ourselves as well as others.

The fifth chakra is known as the Vishuddha (purity) Chakra. This chakra is associated with our throat and thyroid. This governs our general well being and outward personality. If it is open freely we always feel positive and confident in expressing ourselves to others.

The sixth Chakra is known as the Ajna (command) chakra. This chakra is associated with our pineal gland and brain. We have to train ourselves to full activate this chakra. This chakra governs our will power and self-worth. It helps us to follow our thoughts, ideas and practices wilfully.

Biorhythms, Breath Cycles and The Swara

Breathing is one of the involuntary functions in our body, where we don't have much will or consciousness. Breathing is simply an autonomic function governed by our autonomic nervous system. It is a biological function keeping us alive, but still we take it almost for granted. Once we start to know a little about Swaras and study the biorhythmic changes of our body and mind that we go through everyday, we begin to understand how much role our Swaras or nostrils are playing in our psychological, physiological, biological, and hormonal changes to help us to wake up, rest, sleep, eat, digest, act, and think in so many ways.

You will be amazed to find that most of the time we predominantly breath through the right or left nostril. Swara Yoga explains that each nostril or Swara stays open for a period of one Ghatika known as 48 minutes in the scriptures. Breath flowing in left nostril is known as Chandra Swara, while breath flowing in right nostril is known as Surya Swara. These Swara cycles alternate throughout everyday, every one to two hours. These cycles alternate in a rhythm throughout the day and night. This pattern or change is also deeply connected with the moon or lunar cycles.

Each afternoon around sun set our left nostril dominates to prepare our body and mind for sleep, while around sunrise our right nostril dominates to prepare our body and mind for waking up. At the end of each cycle our breath flows equally or freely through both nostrils for 1 to 3 minutes. In this period our energy flows into Sushumna Nadi and there is sense of balance and inner peace.

Around the 1970s the word 'chrono-psychology' was given for the study and understanding of the 24 hour cycle of physical and psychological changes we all go through everyday. These Chrono-Psychologists found that, "In a 24 hour cycle, most people go through certain biological events and changes and one's mental, emotional and physical abilities have a 'best' or 'most favourable' time of the day". Swara yoga details the same, but even further, on when and how to perform various daily life activities as well as how to manipulate these energetic biorhythmic changes to enhance our life and energy.

Chronopsychology is a discipline that studies mechanisms and functions of rhythmicity in psychological variables such as memory, perception and emotional processes.

These ancient teachings of Swara yoga also perfectly align with the findings of our modern neurophysiologists and neuroanatomists. These investigations of our brain details that our brain doesn't function as a single unit. Our brain functions as a combination of two bilateral hemispheres known as right and left brain. These two parts are connected with a thin membrane. The nerve fibers corpus callosum separates the right and left half of the brain.

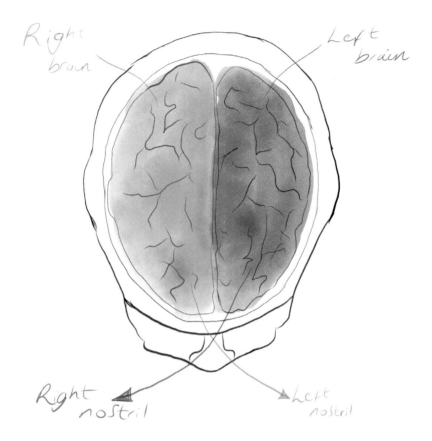

The right side of the brain governs the functions of the left side of the body. Also the right side of our brain governs the left nostril breathing and vice-versa the left nostril breathing stimulates the right brain through stimulation of nerves endings in the left nostril areas. This is similarly explained as the Ida or Chandra Swara in Swara yoga. Conversely, the left hemisphere of our brain controls the right side our our body. This stimulates right nostril breathing or Pingala Nadi and Surya Swara. Modern research also shows that our right nostril breath stimulates our left brain and left nostril breathing stimulates our right brain.

According to neurophysiologists, our brain actually switches alternatively between the left and right hemispheres in every 60-90 minutes likewise Swara yoga teachings. It further mentions that at the end of each cycle, nerve impulses or energy are discharged in the nerve fibres corpus callosum for around 4 minutes. These findings tremendously correspond with the Swara cycles, the period and even the time of changes and flow of energy in Sushumna Nadi for 1-3 minutes.

If we look further, then the active right or left side of brain also stimulate the corresponding nostril into operation. This explains how one nostrils remains open while other one is partially blocked. This gives us a little understanding of Swaras from the scientific perspective.

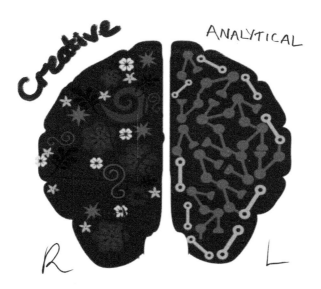

There are also findings that during the first half of these cycles, the energy gradually builds up to a peak potential, which lead our body and mind to high alertness and sensitivity. In the second part the energy gradually declines. People with chromic illness suffer or undergo pain and disturbed energy in the first half of the cycle.

These findings can even explain how we behave, act, react and respond to similar events so differently at different parts of even the same day. This explains the links of our brain with our breath and the way we think, feel and perceive different events throughout the day. This is something that is explained in Samkhya Yoga and Bhagavat Gita that our soul is not doing any of our karma, and neither taking part in any of our actions, it neither consumes any of the fruits. Our soul or Atman is not a doer - Karta, neither perceiver - Drastha and neither consumer - Bhokta'. This phenomena explains that all our physical, mental and emotional activities and choices are derived or governed by these energetic changes and the dominance of one or other parts of the brain. Krishna says in Bhagavat Gita that all our Karmas are taking place under the guiding force of Tri-Gunas and Prakriti or inherited nature or life governing energy. We are just acting, reacting and responding according to the pre-programmed cosmic biorhythmic energy cycles and brain.

The Yoga Chudamani Upanishad, describes "the Jiva or individual consciousness is governed by the action of the breath". The Hatha Yoga Pradipika (4:21) mentions that: "He who has mastered his breath has also mastered the fields of the mind and by mastering the mental one also masters the breath."

Swara yoga scriptures further details the effect or influence of moon cycles on our Swaras or Nostrils. Shukla Paksha is 15 days long including the waxing moon period. Krishna Paksha also includes 15 days if waning moon. Tithis is like the day of the month or date in our English calendar. Here is the table of Swaras with the moon calendar from Swara Yoga.

Swaras and Lunar Cycles

Days	Tithis	Fort nigh;	Sunrise	Sunset swara
1	Pratipada	Shukla Paksha	Ida (left nostril)	Pingala (right nostril)
2	Dwitiya	Shukla Paksha	Ida	Pingala
3	Tritiya	Shukla Paksha	Ida	Pingala
4	Chaturthi.	Shukla Paksha	Pingala	Ida
5	Panchami	Shukla Paksha	Pingala	Ida
6	Shashthi	Shukla Paksha	Pingala	Ida
7	Saptami.	Shukla Paksha	Ida	Pingala
8	Ashtami.	Shukla Paksha	Ida	Pingala
9	Navami.	Shukla Paksha	Ida	Pingala
10	Dashami.	Shukla Paksha	Pingala	Ida

11	Ekadasi.	Shukla Paksha	Pingala	Ida
12	Dwadashi.	Shukla Paksha	Pingala	Ida
13	Trayodashi.	Shukla Paksha	Ida	Pingala
14	Chaturdashi.	Shukla Paksha	Ida	Pingala
15	Purnima	Full moon	Ida	Pingala
16	Pratipada	Krishna Paksha	Pingala	Ida
17	Dwitiya	Krishna Paksha	Pingala	Ida
18	Tritiya	Krishna Paksha	Pingala	Ida
19	Chaturthi.	Krishna Paksha	Ida	Pingala
20	Panchami	Krishna Paksha	Ida	Pingala
21	Shashthi	Krishna Paksha	Ida	Pingala
22	Saptami.	Krishna Paksha	Pingala	Ida
23	Ashtami.	Krishna Paksha	Pingala	Ida
24	Navami.	Krishna Paksha	Pingala	Ida
25	Dashami.	Krishna Paksha	Ida	Pingala

26	Ekadasi.	Krishna Paksha	Ida	Pingala
27	Dwadashi.	Krishna Paksha	Ida	Pingala
28	Trayodashi.	Krishna Paksha	Pingala	Ida
29	Chaturdashi.	Krishna Paksha	Pingala	Ida
30	Amawashya	No Moon	Pingala	Ida

Modern science has revealed the relation of our breath, nostrils, brain and mind, but they have not got as far as Swara yoga science so far; to explore the Nadis, breath cycles and their relation with lunar and solar cycles. Pawan Vijaya Swarodaya details how our Swaras, Nadis or Nostrils are active at sunrise and sunset with the lunar cycles from waxing to waning moon.

Synchronise the Swara for Better Health

If the Chandra or Suriya Swaras or right and left Swara are not aligned with the solar or lunar cycles, then one can consciously manipulate the Swaras to synchronise the Swaras for better health and well-being as well as intoning with biorhythms. Here are some simple practices to change the Swara:-

Regular practice of Jala Neti and Sutra Neti to cleanse your nostrils will help remove any physical blockage. Close the free flowing nostril and breathe in and out through the inactive nostril for a few minutes. Inhale through the dominating nostril and exhale through the dormant nostril as Suriya or Chandra Nadi Pranayama for 3 to 5 minutes.

Apply pressure to the armpit on the same side as the active nostril. You may use the fist of the opposite hand and place it inside the armpit and hold the pressure. After some time the opposite nostril will become activated. This is why Yogis always kept a Danda or stick to rest the armpit for changing the nostrils in Yoga Ashrams or traditions.

Lay on the active nostril side of the body to change the nostril to the opposite side with head resting on folded arm and upper leg also fold with the knee on the floor in front with the foot resting behind the opposite knee. These postures are known as Surya and Chandra Nadi Asanas. So if you want to change nostril from right to left then lie on your right side with left side dominating.
The external environment also influences nasal activity. Washing the body or just the face with hot or cold water automatically changes the breath flow.

The type of food consumed will affect the Nadis. Foods which heat the body, will stimulate Surya Nadi, while foods that cool the system, will activate Chandra Nadi.

Counterbalancing the over active Nadi for Health

Our physical and mental health can be understood by knowing the Swara cycles or nostril alternation cycles in our daily life. If one of the Nadi remains active for too long, it will cause strain on particular areas of the nervous system, especially the autonomic nervous system. This will over stress those nerves being over stimulated as well as the associated part of brain. This will imbalance our body and mind as one half of our being is over active while the other half will be under active. It will affect our homeostasis and healing process.

Once we can understand the relation of our Swara with body parts, energy and associated functions, we can establish the relation of over and under active Nadis with various health issues. By switching the nostrils regularly we help healing in many of these health issues.

When the Ida Nadi or Swara is over active, we are lacking the fire or Pranic heating energy. This will result in poor digestion, flatulence, indigestion, diarrhoea, dysentery, cholera, and dyspepsia. Also further respiratory problems, lack of energy, and life drive can be associated with this too.

When the Pingala Nadi or Swara is over active, we suffer with stress related problems like hypertension, acidity, ulcers, emotional instability, anger, etc.

According to Shiva Swarodaya we can enhance a good, healthy and long life by maximising the flow of the Ida Swara during the day and the flow of the Pingala Nadi during the night time. This counterbalances the over activation of heating solar breathing in day and cooling lunar energy in the night time. In the night time we should always try to go to sleep on the left side with the right side dominating in Suriya Nadi Asana. Many of us suffer with so many health issues just because of lack of proper deep sleep.

As a curative or rehabilitation tool, these Swara Yoga tools can be used for a holistic healing process. You will find that people with digestive problems tend to sleep more on their right side. Resting more often on the left side can help rectify many digestion issues. Similarly people with breathing disorders tend to sleep more their backs. Asthmatic people can benefit more by sleeping on the left side and activating Surya or Pingala Swara to activate heating energy.

We can bring body temperature down by sleeping on the right side or activating Ida Swara and raise the body temperature up by sleeping on the left side or activating Pingala Swara. Ida Swara will help in relieving hypertension while Pingala Swara will help in relieving hypo-tension. So simply by switching the Swara or energy flow, we will counterbalance our body and mind and gradually attain harmony and balance.

Even before we see the symptoms of any health issues, we can notice the disturbance in the cycles of Swara or nostril changes. If we can notice this or can be mindful, then we just need to change the nostrils or Swara to prevent the sickness or lessen the severity of a health problem.

Pranayama and Swara Yoga

Yoga guides on how to unite and balance the two opposing forces of Loma-Viloma, Prana-Apana, Surya-Chandra, Ida-Pingala or positive-negative energies to live in harmony and balance. Yoga is also known as harmony and living in equanimity. Swara Yoga teaches us some of the Kriyas and Prakriyas as well as how to manipulate our nostrils and Swaras to balance and harmonise our energies.

The Hatha Yoga Pradipika explains Surya and Chandra Nadi Pranayama, and Nadi Sodhana Pranayama to balance these energies and directly stimulate or activate the right and left brains. It further mentions that by balancing our energy, we can balance our whole body and live in health and harmony.

The Hatha Yoga Pradipika in chapter two mentions, "A Sadhaka should inhale through the left nostril and retain the breath. Follow this by expelling the breath through the right nostril. Now inhale through the right nostril and retain the breath. Exhale through the left nostril for purification of our Nadi system". This is known as Nadi Sodhana Pranayama. This means the Swara Yoga Sadhana involves the Pranayama Sadhana.

Swara is linked with the breath and so does the Prana. So breath becomes the tool for a Pranayama and Swara Yoga Sadhaka. Still we should not misunderstand Swara Yoga as Pranayama like many people understand Pranayama as breathing exercises. Breath is merely a tool for Pranayama Sadhana. Pranayama aims to enhance the Prana energy and use that for purification, rejuvenation and awakening. Swara Yoga uses the nature of inhalation and exhalation and the cycles of nostril change and learning to manipulate them for balance and harmony.

Daily Reading of the Breath and Swara

We spend so much time on reading news, watching television, which contribute very little to our health and evolution. In reverse these may drain so much of our energy and create so much negativity, unnecessary desires and fear. Swara Yoga advises us to read our nostrils or Swara daily. All we have to do is just relax and notice which nostril we are breathing dominantly with and note it down. As part of Yogic diagnosis for Swara Yoga Therapy we need at least a good week or so of daily nostril reading. Try to make a chart of a week of Swara reading around sunrise and sunset time daily. According to Swara Yoga each our breath is a sign of our past, present and future at physical, mental, emotional and spiritual levels.

Here are the practices to read the nostril or Swara:

Relax and bring the palm of your one hand in front of your nose. Exhale your breath and notice which nostril is expelling a strong current of air; that will be your active nostril.

You can close one of the nostrils and check the flow of breath through the other nostril. You will notice it will be easier to inhale and exhale through one nostril compared to other. The easier nostril will be the active Swara at that time.

The third method of checking the Swara is by listening to the sound of your breath. An open nostril will have the deeper pitched sound of breath compare to the blocked Swara.

Here as we reading the nostril, we also need to keep in mind the cycle or natural flow or cycle of the Ida and Pingala Swaras, before we learn or practice the manipulation or transformation of Swaras.

Living in Harmony with the Swaras

We have already discussed the particular times and cycles of Nadis and Swaras and how to change them if needed. Now we need to understand the relation of Swaras with various daily activities and events of life. When a particular Swara is active, particular areas of brain and body are also predominantly active compared to the opposite parts. This should give us some idea of the influence of our nostril or Swara on our body and mind and the activities associated with them.

According to Sperry's research, the left brain is associated with:

- logic
- sequencing
- linear thinking
- mathematics
- facts
- thinking in words

The right brain is more visual and intuitive. It's sometimes referred to as the analog brain. It has a more creative and less organised way of thinking.

Sperry's research suggests the right brain is associated with:

- imagination
- holistic thinking
- intuition
- arts

- rhythm
- nonverbal cues
- feelings visualisation
- daydreaming

Source-https://embryo.asu.edu/pages/roger-sperrys-split-brain-experiments-1959-1968

The Swara Yoga mentions that when our Ida Nadi or Chandra Swara is active, which means the right hemisphere or part of the brain is active too, we have access to vibration realms of existence, which is not subject to our sensory perception. All information and experiences in this field are processed in a widely spread field of experience. Our abilities of creativity, imaginative and intuitive fields are at an enhanced level.

IDA	PINGALA
Left nostril	Right nostril
Right hemisphere	Left hemisphere
Introversion	Extroversion
Mental and artistic work	Physical and dynamic work
Metabolism slows down - cool	Metabolism speeds up - warm
Interprets emotional connotation of communication	Use and meaning of words and language, both spoken and written
Recognition of facial expressions	
Intuitive, integrative, accurate	Rational decisions, thinking judgment
Music and art awareness, imagination	Logical, verbal, mathematical, analytical
Perception of space, patterns, direction	

Parasympathetic Nervous System	Sympathetic Nervous System
Management of:	Management of:
- epilepsy	
- obsessive compulsive disorder	- glaucoma.
- high blood pressure	- low blood pressure

Source for the above table- http://www.yogamag.net/archives/2011/joct11/swara2.shtml by Dr Swami Mudraroopa Saraswati

Swara Yoga explains that in our day to day life to enhance our abilities and to live our full potential, we can read our Swara or nostril and then do the suitable activities according to which fields of our body and mind are active or change the nostril or Swara before performing various activities. Swara Yoga explains the suitable Swara for drinking water, eating food, sleeping, waking up, reading, meditation, travelling, doing various tasks or work, etc. Further Swara Yoga details the appropriate Swara for Yoga Sadhana, Mantra chanting, Satsanga and companionship of Guru and the initiation of new activities or business opportunities in life.

The right side, or the Pingala Nadi or Swara is associated with the left side of the brain. Here we process all the information and experiences in a sequence, in a logical and analytical manner. The left hemisphere, stimulated by the right nostril dominance, is connected to masculine, solar, rational verbal and more energetic activities. Our mathematical and rational abilities are at the best in this energy field. Here, energy and awareness are extroverted, hence all the mechanical and physical tasks can be accomplished. When the Pingala or Suriya Swara is active, we have the heating and energetic principles of outgoing and performing physical activity, dynamic performances, and challenging ventures can be performed. All the intellectual work, eating and digestion, extrovert activities and work, and for men, engaging in sexual pleasure can be considered during this energy active period.

The right hemisphere, stimulated by left nostril dominance, is connected to the feminine, lunar, emotional, visual and more peaceful activities.

When the breath flows freely through both the nostrils in a balanced manner, our Sushumna and balanced Swara is active. This is the time to do things where you need the least mental and physical effort. This is a favourable time for spiritual or Adhyatmic Sadhaka and activities. Great Yogis and Rishis seek to induce and prolong the activation and flow of energy upward through this central channel of Sushumna. When the energy or Prana flows for longer durations in Sushumna, Sadhaka experiences higher states of consciousness. A Sadhaka can attain absolute liberation through activating, and flowing the Pranic energy in this channel and this is why Tantra and Swara Yoga emphasise this path.

A few recommendations from Swara Yoga for attuning with our Potential.

Once we have learned how to read and manipulate our Swara or nostril, it's time to learn some basic practices to attune with our biorhythmic energies and enhance our abilities and life forces to attain our highest potential in daily life. These are simple steps we can easily introduce in our daily life.

1. At the time of waking, read your nostrils and check which Swara is active. Now touch the active nostril and that side

of the face with the corresponding hand and take a few conscious breaths.

2. When you step out of the bed, and place the corresponding foot to the active nostril on the earth first. If your Pingala Swara is active, place the right foot on floor first at the time you leave your bed and place the left foot first when your Ida Swara is active.

3. This further says if you are travelling towards the east or north, make sure your Pingala Swara is active and you place the right foot forward first for a successful journey.

4. If you travelling due south or west, make sure your Ida Swara is active and you place your left foot forward first for successful journey.

5. When you are going on an important journey, meeting or task, always step out of your house with the corresponding foot to active nostril.

6. For successful negotiations, business meetings, conflict resolutions, start your approach to these people with first stepping forward the corresponding foot to the active nostril. Further keep your inactive nostril side towards that person during your meeting.

7. If you are receiving or giving something to others, use the hand corresponding to the active nostril.

The Tattwas or Elements in Swara Yoga

Samkhya Yoga explains that in the process of creation, five elements or Pancha-Tattwas are evolutes of Prana, Prakriti and Parmatman. Further all living and non-living material is created from various combinations and the union of these five primary elements, some times also known as Pancha-Mahabhutas. These are; Prathvi or earth, Jala or water, Vayu or air, Agni or fire and Akash space or voidness.

Swara Yoga Sadhana involves two key practices and one of them is Tattwa Sadhana. Swara Yogis explain how to analyse the breath and the relationship of the breath with the inherent Tattwas -earth, water, air, heat and voidness. Swara Yoga details the Mandala or geometric shapes for each of these elements and guides us on Pranayama and Trataka or gazing practices for balancing these Tattwas for physical, mental, emotional and spiritual aligning, balance or harmony. These practices further explain the Yantra and breathing patterns and also their association with the Chakras.

The Second Practice of Swara Yoga Sadhana is known as Chhayopasana, which means Trataka or gazing or focussing our mind on our own shadow. Chhaya is a Sanskrit meaning shadow and Upasana means mastering the practice or Sadhana. Tratak means 'gazing focus'. Trataka can be visual with our eyes, or Trataka can be Manasik or mental with the eyes closed. In these practices, Sadhaka becomes fully aware or focused on the object of attention and transcends from all other sensory and mental distractions. This leads a Sadhaka to attain the inherent wisdom that is coded in each and every manifestation in our universe. These Sadhana practices help develop focus, will power and lead us to experience higher or meditative states of consciousness. This also awakens the subtle and psychic realms or fields of wisdom that are stored in the subtlest of our higher or cortex fields in the brain, as well as in the Chakras, Pranic field and wisdom body or Vijnanamaya Kosha.

Samkhya and Vedas explain that the subtlest of knowledge of creation, life processes, and events are pre-recorded and through mastering these Sadhanas or practices one can have access to these teachings or wisdom. Some scriptures call it Akashik Vijnana or Astral Teachings. One can also experience three Kalas - past, present and future.

The macro and micro-cosmos, Tattwas and Breath

Samkhya Yoga Philosophy on creation details that our universe (macro-cosmos) is created from the composition of five subtle primordial elements, known as earth, water, air, fire and ether or voidness. Similarly our body (micro-cosmos) is also composed from these same elements and our bodies are representative of models of the whole universe. Our body has the information or wisdom of the whole universe coded in each and every cell. Swara yoga details that these elements are hidden behind each and every living and non-living material and by knowing the breath, we can also know or experience or decode the knowledge of the universe. This nature or universe and quality of elements can be understood by knowing the exhaling breath. Taittriya Upanishad mentions that by focussing on the five Tattwas, the various elements and the way the materials manifest can be known.

Further Samkhya Yoga, the Mandukya-Upanishad, Prashna-Upanishad and Shiva Swarodaya explain that the five Tattwas are evolutes of Supreme Consciousness. Prana Evolutes from Divine Consciousness or Parmatman. Mind manifests from Prana and Pancha-Mahabhutas or these five elements are evolutes of the mind. These Tattwas are subject to our sensory experience and hence by focusing our mind on each of the Tattwa, we can expand our awareness and experience higher or supreme consciousness.

How to Read the Tattwas

Like the Swara, the state of body and mind and lunar and solar energy affect our breathing and energy, it is also connected with which element or Tattwa is predominantly active at this point. We can understand that by measuring the length of our breath. Here is the table:-

Element	Earth	Water	Fire	Air	Ether
Length in fingers	12	16	4	8	-
Length in inches	9	12	3	6	-
Direction	centre	downwards	upwards	slanting	diffused
Duration (minutes)	1st	2nd	3rd	4th	5th
Sequence	1st	2nd	3rd	4th	5th

Manifestations of the elements

These Tattwas can be gross or subtle in nature and all the living and non-living materials in the universe manifest from these five elements. The nature and qualities of each and every material will depend on the composition of these five elements and ratios or sequence of the activeness. These properties create our macro and micro-cosmos. Shiva Swarodaya mentions that all the changes and transformations are taking place due to these elements. Here is the table of various characteristics and representations of these Tattwas-

Element	Prithvi	Jala	Agni	Vayu	Akash
Nature	heavy	Cool	Warmth	unpredictable	mixed
Quality	Solid	Liquid	Heat	Wind	Void
Color	yellow	white	red	grey or blue	mixture (blackish)
Shape	Square	Crescent moon	Triangle	Pentagon	Bindu
Chakra	mooladhara	swadhisthana	manipura	anahata	vishuddhi
Mantra	Lam	Vam	Ram	Yam	Ham
Tanmatra	Smell	Taste	Sight	Touch	Sound
States of mind	ego (ahamkara)	intellect (buddhi)	mind (manas)	Self or consciousness (chitta)	cosmic consciousness (mahat)
Kosha	Annamaya	Pranamaya	Manomaya	Vijnanamaya	Anandamaya
Place in body	Below knees	Anal area to thighs	Anal area to heart	heart to third eye area	Above third eye
Function in body	skin, veins & arteries, skeleton	fluids in the body	appetite, thirst, sleep	Contraction-extension of muscles, movement	emotions and passions
Planet	Venus	Mercury	Mars	Saturn	Jupiter
Direction	east	west	south	north	Upward

We can check the active Tattwa by taste or flavour in the mouth after a few hours of fasting. Earth element is sweetish, water is salty, fire is hot or pungent, air is acidic or sour and ether is bitter in flavour.

You can also expel your breath through your nose onto a clean mirror and try to read the pattern of the vapour. If the earth element is active, vapour will cover the mirror, while a half moon shape indicates water, triangular shapes represent fire, an oval shape indicates air and small dots indicate ether or voidness as the active element.

The third way to find out which Tattwa is predominantly active is by practicing Shanmukhi or Yoni Mudra. Use your hands to close all the orifices of eyes, ears, nose and lips with your fingers and focus your mind on inner light known as Anter-Jyoti behind the eyebrow centre. Gradually you may see a coloured circle. A Yellow colour indicates activation of earth Tattwa, white represents the water element, red represents fire, blue or grey represent air and black represents ether or voidness.

Mandala dharana and Maldala Pranayama for Tattwa Sadhana

Once we are able to know which Tattwa is active, we can understand the significance and life energy flows to attain our true potential in day to day life.

When the Prathvi Tattwa is active, it is suitable to perform stable, and calm activities. A good time for Mantra Chanting, Pranayama and meditation practices as Yoga Sadhana. This is a great time to undertake new opportunities and tasks to be fruitful.

When water or Jala Tattwa is active, it is a good time for movement, transformation and a change of flow. It's a good time to undertake physical and mental work where lots of movement and activity is required. This element bring far less fruits than you may anticipate, as its influence brings moderate fruits.

The fire or Agni Tattwa leads to loss and damage and hence avoid taking physical or mental work in this period where stability and mindfulness is required. It's a great time to perform work and tasks requiring dynamic activities.

When the air or Vayu Tattwa is active, you may expect more negative than positive fruits. It's time where we are unstable and suffer with mental and emotional imbalance. This is a good time for travelling and adventures.

While the ether, voidness or Akash Tattwa is active, it is recommended to perform spiritual activities as all other activities may lead us to failure.

Each of these Tattwa will have different results during the activation of Surya or Chandra Swara.

While the earth and water elements are active, it is auspicious and favourable to perform and undertake any task during the flow of the Ida or Pingala Nadi.

The fire and the air elements are auspicious during the Ida flow. The ether or Akash elements will only be fruitful in spiritual and transcendental practices and will not bring any material fruits.

So, once we understand some of these ideas, we can plan our life events and activities like a surfer organising the time to go for surfing whilst knowing the tides. Further Swara yoga details Tattwa Sadhana practices to change the energy, Swara and Tattwas to live our lives in better harmony with our biorhythms and life events.

The ultimate goal of Swara yoga or Tattwa Sadhana is to connect with our breath, energy flows, subtle elements to know our true nature, and the qualities which leads us to absolute realisation and Samadhi or blissful state.

For Tattwa and Mandala Sadhanas you will need a Guru or teacher to prepare you and take you through each of these practices. You can draw the Mandalas for each element as described in the Sadhana process below.

Recommended Preparation:
1.   Loma-viloma group of asanas
2.   Oli mudras
3.   Loma-viloma and aloma-viloma pranayama

1. Swadhisthana Chakra

Element	**Water**
Mandala shape	**Silvery crescent moon on white**

Draw this Mandala on a clear white sheet and chose a comfortable room. Room should be well ventilated, with light not too bright or dark.

Sit straight tin comfortable meditation posture and hands in Jnana or Dhyana Mudra.

Focus your gaze on the mandalas for a minute or two and then close you eyes and try to visualise the mandala around your Swadhisthana or sacral area for 2 to 3 minutes. Repeat this three times in beginning.

Gradually one can increase this time. With the eyes closed you don't need to force or to try to perceive anything. Try to visualise and allow the natural process to happen inside with your eyes closed.

2. Manipura chakra

Element   **Agni**

Mandala shape   **Red reverse triangle on white sheet**

Draw this Mandala on a clear white sheet and chose a comfortable room. Room should be well ventilated, with light not too bright or dark.

Sit straight tin comfortable meditation posture and hands in Jnana or Dhyana Mudra.

Focus your gaze on the mandalas for a minute or two and then close you eyes and try to visualise the mandala around your Manipura or solar area for 2 to 3 minutes. Repeat this three times in beginning.

Gradually one can increase this time. When you have your eyes closed you don't need to force or try to perceive anything. Try to allow the natural process inside with closed eyes.

3. Anahata chakra

Element   **Air**
Mandala shape   **Two blue triangles intersected on a white sheet**

Draw this Mandala on a clear white sheet and chose a comfortable room. Room should be well ventilated, with light not too bright or dark.

Sit straight tin comfortable meditation posture and hands in Jnana or Dhyana Mudra.

Focus your gaze on the mandalas for a minute or two and then close you eyes and try to visualise the mandala around your Anahata or heart area for 2 to 3 minutes. Repeat this three times in beginning. Gradually one can increase this time. When your eyes are closed you don't need to force or try to perceive anything. Allow the natural process inside with closed eyes.

4. Mooladhara Chakra

Element	Prithvi, Earth
Mandala shape	**Yellow Square in 2d and cube in 3d on white sheet**

Draw this Mandala on a clear white sheet and chose a comfortable room. Room should be well ventilated, with light not too bright or dark.

Sit straight tin comfortable meditation posture and hands in Jnana or Dhyana Mudra.

Focus your gaze on the mandalas for a minute or two and then close you eyes and try to visualise the mandala around your Mooladhara or root area for 2 to 3 minutes. Repeat this three times in beginning. Gradually one can increase this time. When you have the eyes closed you don't need to force or try to perceive anything. Try to visualise the natural process described below with closed eyes.

5. Vishuddha Chakra

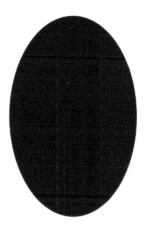

Element   **Akasha, space, ether**
Mandala shape   **Magenta coloured oval shape**

Draw this Mandala on a clear white sheet and chose a comfortable room. Room should be well ventilated, with light not too bright or dark.

Sit straight tin comfortable meditation posture and hands in Jnana or Dhyana Mudra.

Focus your gaze on the mandalas for a minute or two and then close you eyes and try to visualise the mandala around your Vishuddha or throat area for 2 to 3 minutes. Repeat this three times in beginning.

Gradually one can increase this time. When your eyes are closed you don't need to force or try to perceive anything. Try to visualise the natural process described below with closed eyes.

6. Ajna Chakra

Element   **Manas, mind**
Mandal shape   **Orange coloured circle shape**

Draw this Mandala on a clear white sheet and chose a comfortable room. Room should be well ventilated, with light not too bright or dark.

Sit straight tin comfortable meditation posture and hands in Jnana or Dhyana Mudra.

Focus your gaze on the mandalas for a minute or two and then close you eyes and try to visualise the mandala around your Ajna or third eye area for 2 to 3 minutes. Repeat this three times in beginning.

Gradually one can increase this time. When you have your eyes closed you don't need to force or try to perceive anything. Try to visualise the natural process inside with closed eyes.

Chhaya-Upasana, or Shadow Gazing

The most advanced and significant Sadhana or Practice in Swara yoga is Chhaya-Upasana or shadow gazing. Shiva Swarodaya mentions 7- 8am is most suitable time for this Sadhana. Stand in Samsthiti with your back facing the sun and focus your mind on the neck of your own shadow. With the gaze repeat the Mantra 'Hrim Para-Brahmane Namah'. After 9 rounds of Mantra Chanting focus your eyes into the sky and visualise an enhanced version of your own shadow.

You can begin this Sadhana with chanting the Mantra 9 times and gradually increase the chants in multiples of 9 every 9 days. This Sadhana can lead you to super-conscious and extra-sensory perceptions and a transcendent experience.

This is simple, but one of the most advanced Dharna or concentration practices, which leads a Sadhaka to Dhyana or meditation and eventually Samadhi or absolute liberation. This will certainly bring self-realisation or Atmanubhuti. This Sadhana needs sincere preparation of our body, mind, and Nadis through Hatha Yoga, Pranayama, and Jnana Yoga practices under the guidance of a Guru.

Resources and References :-

1. Yoga Step By Step by Dr Swamiji Gitananda Giriji

2. https://www.swarayoga.org/ -articles on Swara yoga by Mukti Bodhananda

3. https://en.wikipedia.org/wiki/Shiva_Swarodaya_/_Swara_Yoga

4. http://www.yogamag.net/

5. Shiva Svarodaya translated by Satyananda Saraswati,1983

6. Shiva Svarodaya Text With English Translation Ram Kumar Rai

7. Swarodaya Vigjnana :-Scientific Analysis of the Nasal Cycle and its Applications by Dr Ananda Balayogi Bhavanani

8. Mukti Bodhananda, 1999 Swara Yoga, Nesma Books India

9. Satyananda Saraswati, 1999 Swara Yoga, Nesma Books India

10. Mukti Bodhananda, 1984, "Swara yoga: the tantric science of brain breathing", Bihar School of Yoga

11. https://www.lifepositive.com/the-almighty-breath/ By Prema Nirmal

12. https://www.ncbi.nlm.nih.gov/pmc/articles/PMC4728953/ By Karamjit Singh, Hemant Bhargav, and TM Srinivasan

13. https://www.ncbi.nlm.nih.gov/pmc/articles/PMC3681046/ By Anant Narayan Sinha, Desh Deepak, and Vimal Singh Gusain

14. http://sequencewiz.org/2014/08/06/one-nostril-breathing/ BY OLGAKABEL

15. https://www.mindbodygreen.com/0-12936/3-reasons-everyone-should-try-alternate-nostril-breathing.html – Dr. Paula Watkins

16. https://chopra.com/articles/nadi-shodhana-how-to-practice-alternate-nostril-breathing – By Melissa Eisler

SWARODAYA VIGJNAN: YOGIC AND SCIENTIFIC UNDERSTANDING OF THE NASAL CYCLE

Yogacharya

Dr ANANDA BALAYOGI BHAVANANI, MD, DSc (Yoga)
Chairman and Hereditary Trustee: International Centre
for Yoga Education & Research (ICYER) at Ananda Ashram,
Puducherry, India. www.icyer.com

INTRODUCTION

Yoga is the evolutionary process of integration (yuj = union). In the Bhagavad Gita, Lord Krishna says "Samatvam yoga uchyate"(Yoga is equanimity). The Yogic concept of Loma Viloma (balancing the dwandwas / opposites) encompasses the wide variety of processes in our body, emotions and mind and thus brings about this equanimity of the mind. Yoga and Tantra emphasize the balance between the two halves of the body in terms of Loma and Viloma. The right side of the body is considered to be of masculine nature, endowed with warm, golden, positive, pranic energy and represented by the pingala nadi (energy channel on the right of the sushumna). The left side of the body is considered feminine and endowed with cool, silvery, negative, apanic energy and represented by the ida nadi (energy channel on the left of the sushumna).

The sushumna nadi is the energy channel that runs down the middle of the central canal of the spinal cord. (Note: All these energy channels are in the pranamaya kosha though they have correlating structures in the physical body).

The Yogin attempts to understand, harness and bring about a balance between the energies of the two halves of the body. The best practical example of this concept is found in the study of the nasal cycle.

The nasal cycle is an ultradian rhythm of nasal congestion and decongestion with a quasi-periodicity of 60 to 240 minutes. Keyser made the first formal description and the use of the term nasal cycle in 1895. However the concept of the nasal cycle and an understanding of its role in our life had existed for long before that in Indian thought.

The Vedic science of understanding the function of the nasal cycle was known as Swarodaya Vigjnan (swara = sonorous sound produced by the airflow through the nostrils in the nasal cycle, udaya = functioning state, and vigjnan = knowledge). The Shivaswarodaya, an ancient treatise in Sanskrit literature advises the Yogi to undertake quieter, passive activities (soumya karya) when the left nostril flow is dominant (ida / chandra swara), to engage in challenging and exertional activities (roudra karya) when right nostril is dominant (pingala / surya swara) and to relax or meditate when the bilateral nasal flow is operational (sushumna swara) as it was considered to be unsuitable for performance of worldly activities.

Ida swara (left nostril dominance) was described as feminine, Shakti and moon-like (chandra) while the pingala swara (right nostril dominance) was described as masculine, Shiva and sun-like (surya).

Similarly the traditional Indian description of Ardhanarishwara consists of Shakti (the female element) being depicted on the left and Shiva (the male element) on the right side of the body.

Such a notion of left-right, female-male duality was common in oriental traditional medicine as also in western alchemy. The nasal cycle has been demonstrated not only in man but also in rat, rabbit and domestic pig.

TRADITIONAL VIEWS ON SWARA YOGA

A. Rhythmicity of the swara

Textbooks of swara yoga (Charandas, 1954; Kannan, 1967; Gautam, 1975) describe a definite pattern of breathing in a healthy person on each day of the month at sunrise. It is said that on days 1,2,3,7,8,9,13,14,15 of the bright fortnight (the two weeks after full moon), the breath is to flow predominantly in the left nostril at sunrise and on days 4,5,6,10,11,12 it is to flow in the right nostril at sunrise. Similarly, on days 1,2,3,7,8,9,13,14,15 of the dark fortnight (the two weeks after the new moon), the breath is to flow predominantly in the right nostril at sunrise and on days 4,5,6,10,11,12 it is to flow in the left nostril at sunrise. In modern man it is difficult to have these natural patterns due to the haphazard life styles but in preliminary studies conducted on students attending six months Yoga Training at ICYER, Yogamaharishi Dr. Swami Gitananda had reported a definite relationship between the lunar phase and the swara pattern.

B. Activities prescribed in various swaras

1. Activities prescribed in lunar Swara
   Initiation of new projects, intake of hot liquids, studies and learning, travelling, dancing, singing, weddings and other auspicious ceremonies are prescribed to be performed when in the lunar (left nostril dominant) swara.

2. Activities prescribed in solar swara
   Strenuous activities such as sporting activities, creative writing, commencing of battle, intake of food, sleep and extension of business are prescribed activities to be performed when in the solar (right nostril dominant) swara.

3. Activities prescribed in sushumna swara
   During the time that both nostrils are functioning equally, it is prohibited to perform any worldly activities and the activities advised are Yogabhyasa, meditaion, puja and other such spiritual and relaxing activities.

C. Interesting observations on swara yoga

Some interesting observations that are made in relation to swara yoga are;

1. Major meals should be partaken in the solar swara.
2. Bathing should be performed in the solar swara and there is danger of catching cold if done in the lunar swara.
3. Articles of hot potency should be taken in the lunar swara as also liquids.
4. Articles of cold potency should be taken in solar swara.
5. One should go to sleep in the solar swara.
6. If male partner has solar swara and female partner has lunar swara during coitus, then the child conceived will be male.

The converse would beget a female child (This interesting observation would be worth being studied scientifically).

7. If a person has headache, cold, hypertension, acidity or asthmatic attack, the change of his swara pattern artificially to the opposite swara may benefit and give relief within an hour. (Again this is worth being studied scientifically, as it would be of use in immediate symptomatic benefit for patients found true.)

8. Indulgence in coitus during flow of same swara of both partners will not result in pregnancy. (Worth scientific investigation as it would be a very effective family planning method is found to be true.)

MECHANISM OF NASAL CYCLE

Various mechanisms were postulated for the occurrence of the nasal cycle and a great amount of research work has been done in this field. The teleological explanation indicates that as one nostril was active in its air-conditioning function, the other nostril rested.

It has been seen that the use of Yoga Danda (T-shaped wooden implement used by the Yogis to regulate differential breathing patterns), pressure of a crutch in the axilla, pressure on the thorax while sitting and also the act of lying down on the side all affect the pattern of nasal dominance. All these maneuvers cause decreased airflow in the ipsilateral (same side) nostril and increased airflow in the contra lateral (opposite side) nostril.

The pattern takes a minute to start to change, equalizes in both nostrils by about the 4th minute and reaches the peak in 17 minutes with application of a crutch and 11 minutes by lateral recumbence. Congestion of the mucosa of one nostril leads to the contra lateral nostril becoming dominant and vice versa.

The nasal cycle is dependent upon the tonic activity of the limbic autonomic nervous system, the levels of circulating catecolamines and other neuro-hormones.

Vinod Deshmukh showed that nasal congestion correlates with low sympathetic-high parasympathetic activity whereas decongestion is directly related to high sympathetic-low parasympathetic activity mode. Virendra Singh showed that compression of the hemi thorax from any surface lateral, anterior, posterior or superior could lead to congestion of the ipsilateral nostril with simultaneous decongestion of the opposite nostril. Keuning has demonstrated that anaesthetizing the nose or the larynx does not influence the nasal cycle but that the nasal cycle is absent after cervical sympathetic denervation and laryngectomy. Mitti Mohan and Eccles showed that airflow in the patent and congested nostrils caused reflex congestion of the patent nostril. Eccles also proposed that the hypothalamus was the centre for the sympathetic effects on the nasal mucosa and the nasal cycle.

MECHANISM OF THE NASAL CYCLE

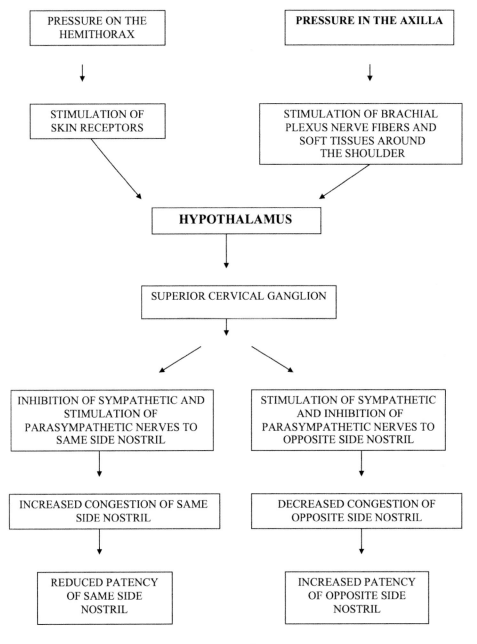

EFFECTS OF NASAL CYCLE AND FORCED UNINOSTRIL BREATHING

Wernitz and others reported selective hemispheric stimulation by unilateral forced breathing. They showed that forced breathing through one nostril produces a relative increase in the EEG amplitude in the contra lateral hemisphere. Block et al demonstrated that unilateral breathing affects males ipsilaterally on both spatial and verbal tasks. Their spatial performance is better during right nostril breathing and verbal performance is better during left nostril breathing. In females it affects performance contra laterally but only in spatial tasks and their spatial performance is better during left nostril breathing. However in a study on 108 school children, K.V Naveen and others found that Yogic breathing through a particular nostril increases spatial rather than verbal scores without lateralised effects.

Swami Gitananda reported that a sensation of well being and good health was experienced by the subjects during the even nostril flows or with right nostril breathing. They also found concentration and meditation to be easier at such times.

Mitti Mohan tested the nostril dominance with reference to the bilateral volar GSR (galvanic skin resistance) that is an indicator of sympathetic activity. He found that sympathetic activity was lower in ida swara, (left nostril breathing) followed by pingala swara (right nostril breathing) and was the maximum in the sushumna swara (bilateral nostril breathing).

Backon has shown that right nostril breathing significantly increases blood glucose levels, whereas left nostril breathing lowers it.

Shirley Telles et all have shown that right nostril breathing can significantly increase the metabolism measured by the increased baseline oxygen consumption with one month of practice several times a day. They have also shown that breathing through the left nostril exclusively, repeated 4 times a day produced a significant increase in the baseline GSR suggestive of reduced sympathetic activity to the palmer sweat glands.

L.Rai et al found that induced left nostril breathing produced decreased systolic, diastolic and mean blood pressures. They suggested that the left nostril breathing could be used as a prophylactic means to combat rises in blood pressure associated with everyday stress and strain of life. They also found that induced right nostril breathing caused correction of blood pressure to normal levels, increase heart rate, increase skin conductance and increased body temperature.

THERAPEUTIC APPLICATIONS OF SWARA YOGA:

A group of pranayama, namely chandra and surya nadi (CN and SN, respectively) and chandra bhedana and surya bhedana (CB and SB, respectively) have uninostril breathing (UNB) and alternate nostril breathing (ANB) patterns using left and/or right nostrils, respectively. This type of Yogic nostril manipulation is also furthered in nadi shuddhi (NS), a specific technique involving alternate use of both nostrils in a specific pattern. It has been previously suggested that right nostril dominance in the nasal cycle as well as right UNB may be correlated with the "activity phase" of the basic rest-activity cycle, the time during which sympathetic activity in general exceeds parasympathetic activity throughout the body. These techniques utilize such knowledge to consciously regulate homeostatic mechanisms of human physiology resulting in beneficial changes. These Yogic UNB and ANB techniques have captured the imagination of researchers worldwide and recent studies have reported their differential physiological and psychological effects. This includes effects on O2 consumption, metabolism and body weight, blood glucose, involuntary blink rates and intraocular pressure, heart rate (HR), stroke volume and end diastolic volume as well as skin resistance, digit pulse volume, and blood pressure (BP).(15) ANB (as done in NS pattern) has been reported to rapidly alter cardiopulmonary responses and improve simple problem solving. Yogic breathing through right, left, or through both nostrils alternately produce distinct autonomic changes: right UNB increased systolic pressure (SP) and diastolic pressure (DP), whereas left UNB resulted in significant reduction in SP and mean pressure (MP).

Shannahoff-Khalsa suggested that mechanical receptors in the nasal mucosa register flow of air across membranes (unilaterally) and transmit this signal ipsilaterally to the hypothalamus, the highest center for autonomic regulation. Alternating left-right levels of catecholamines have been found to occur in peripheral circulation of resting humans with rhythms coupled to the nasal cycle. It is possible that the right nostril initiated techniques are producing such a state of autonomic arousal, whereas left nostril initiated techniques are inducing autonomic relaxation/balance in our subjects.

RESEARCH STUDIES AT CYTER, PONDICHERRY:

Our studies at CYTER, the Centre for Yoga Therapy Education and Research in the Sri Balaji Vidyapeeth (www.sbvu.ac.in/cyter) have demonstrated that right and left yogic UNB and ANB techniques have differential physiological effects. Right nostril initiated UNB and ANB techniques (SB and SN) induce a state of arousal through sympathetic activation and/through increased ascending reticular activity and/or by central action at the primary thalamo-cortical level. On the other hand, left nostril initiated UNB and ANB techniques (CB, CN, NS) delay reactivity of the subjects by inducing a sense of inert lethargy and may induce a state of parasympathetic dominance as manifested in CV parameters. This finding is in tune with the traditional swara yoga concept that air flow through right nostril (SN and pingala swara) is activatory in nature, whereas the flow through left nostril (CN and ida swara) is relaxatory. Further studies in different populations and in patients of different conditions, as well as over different periods of time, may provide a more detailed understanding of the therapeutic potential of these simple and effective pranayama techniques.

CONCLUSION

The science of swara that is of recent interest to scientists all over the world, had been analysed extensively by Indian Yogis of lore. Though they lacked the physical equipment available to modern science, these Yogis through their dedicated practice (abhyasa), inner vision (antar drishti) and self-analysis (swadyaya) had made an extensive number of observations on this concept.

Recent scientific studies have helped us to have a better, methodical understanding of these concepts. They have thrown light on the potential health benefits of forced uninostril breathing in various medical conditions. Further research is required to prove the efficacy of these techniques in clinical conditions such as hypertension, low blood pressure, autonomic dysfunction and diabetes.

The interesting observation that changing the nasal dominance pattern to the opposite side may relieve conditions such as acute asthma, acidity and headache, requires further studies before such techniques can be advocated for clinical trials and patient care.
The theory that conception doesn't occur when both partners are in same swara if found true, will be a welcome addition to the contraceptive armory especially in situations where other methods such as oral contraception are contraindicated.

In conclusion, it can be said that the swara yoga concept is a highly interesting field for further research and it may have wonderful scope in the field of patient care and in improving our understanding of how to live in harmony with nature.

REFERENCES

Backon J. Changes in blood glucose levels induced by differential forced nostril breathing, a technique which affects brain hemisphericity and autonomic activity. Med Sci Res 1988; 16: 1197-99.

Bhavanani AB, Ramanathan M, Balaji R, Pushpa D. Differential effects of uninostril and alternate nostril pranayamas on cardiovascular parameters and reaction time. Int J Yoga 2014; 7: 60-65.

Bhavanani AB, Ramanathan M, Madanmohan. Immediate effect of alternate nostril breathing on cardiovascular parameters and reaction time. Online International Interdisciplinary Research Journal 2014; 4: 297-302.

Bhavanani AB. Swarodaya vigjnan. A scientific study of the nasal cycle. Yoga Mimamsa.2007; 39: 32–38.

Bhole M.V et al. Significance of nostrils in breathing. Yoga Mimamsa 1968; 10(4): 1-12.

Block RA, Arnott DP, Quigley B, Lynch WC. Unilateral nostril breathing influences lateralised cognitive performance. Brain Cognit 1989; 9:181-90.

Davies AM, Eccles R. Reciprocal changes in nasal resistance to air flow caused by pressure applied to the axilla. Acta Otolaryngol (Stockh) 1985; 99:154-59.

Deshmukh VD. Limbic autonomic arousal: its physiological classification and review of the literature. Clinical Electroencephalography 1991; 22: 46-60.

Eccles R. The Central Rhythm of the Nasal Cycle. Acta Oto-Laryngologica 1978; 86: 464-68.

Gitananda Swami. Alternate Pranic flows- A scientific investigation. Yoga Life 2001; 32 (9): 17-18.

Kayser R. Die exakte Messung der Luftdurchgängigkeit der Nase. Arch. Laryng. Rhinol (Berl.) 1895; 3: 101-210.

Kennedy B, Ziegler MG, Shannahoff-Khalsa DS. Alternating lateralization of plasma catecholamines and nasal patency in humans. Life Sci 1986; 38: 1203–14.

Keuning J. On the nasal cycle. Rhinol Int 1968; 6:99-136.

Mitti Mohan S and R Eccles. Effect of inspiratory and expiratory air flow on congestion and decongestion in the nasal cycle. Indian J of Physiol Pharmac 1989; 33: 191-3.

Mitti Mohan S. Reflex reversal of nostril dominance by application of pressure to the axilla by a crutch. Indian J of Physiol Pharmacol 1993; 37(1): 147-50.

Mitti Mohan S. Reversal of nostril dominance by posture. J Indian Med Association 1991; 89:88-91.

Mitti Mohan S. Svara (Nostril dominance) and bilateral volar GSR. Indian J of Physiol Pharmacol 1996; 40(1): 58-64.

Mohan SM, Reddy SC, Wei LY. Modulation of intraocular pressure by unilateral and forced unilateral nostril breathing in young healthy human subjects. Int Ophthalmol 2001;24: 305–11.

Naveen K.V et al. Yoga breathing through a particular nostril increases spatial memory scores without lateralised effects. Psychol Rep 1997; 81(2): 555-61.

Raghuraj P, Telles S. Immediate effect of specific nostril manipulating yoga breathing practices on autonomic and respiratory variables. Appl Psychophysiol Biofeedback 2008; 33: 65–75.

Rai L et al. Effect of induced left nostril breathing on body functions in adult human males. Indian J Physiol Pharmacol 1983(Supplement 1); 5: 74-5.

Rakesh Giri, Ganesh Shankar.Swara Yoga - an introduction and its applications. Nisargopachar Varta 2001; January: 18-20.

Ramanathan M and Bhavanani AB. Immediate effect of chandra and suryanadi pranayamas on cardiovascular parameters and reaction time in a geriatric population. International Journal of Physiology 2014; 2: 59-63.

Rao S, Potdar A. Nasal airflow with body in various positions. J Appl Physiol 1970; 28:162-65.

Shannahoff-Khalsa DS, Kennedy B. The effects of unilateral forced nostril breathing on the heart. Int J Neurosci 1993; 73: 47–60.

Shannahoff-Khalsa DS. Unilateral forced nostril breathing: Basic science, clinical trials, and selected advanced techniques. Subtle Energies and Energy Med J. 2002; 12: 79–106.

Shirley Telles, R Nagaratna and HR Nagendra. Breathing through a particular nostril can alter metabolism and autonomic activities. Indian J Physiol Pharmacol 1994; 38(2): 133-7.

Singh V. Thoracic pressure and nasal patency. J Appl Physiol 1987; 62: 91-94.

Subbalakshmi NK, Saxena SK, Urmimala, D'Souza UJ. Immediate effect of 'Nadi-shodhana Pranayama' on selected parameters of cardiovascular, pulmonary, and higher functions of brain. Thai J Physiol Sci 2005; 18: 10–16.

Telles S, Nagarathna R, Nagendra HR. Breathing through a particular nostril can alter metabolism and autonomic activities. Indian J Physiol Pharmacol 1994; 38: 133–37.

Telles S, Nagarathna R, Nagendra HR. Physiological measures of right nostril breathing. J Altern Complement Med 1996; 2: 479–84.

Vaidya JS, Dhume RA. Influence of lateral posture on sweating: does posture alter the sympathetic outflow to the sweat glands? Indian J Physiol Pharmacol 1994; 38(4): 319-22.

Virendra Singh. Thoracic pressure and nasal patency. J Appl Physiol 1987; 62 (1): 91-94.

Wertz DA, Bickford RG, Shannahkoff-Khalsa D. Selective hemispheric stimulation by uninostril forced nostril breathing. Human Neurobiology 1987; 6:165-71.

Glossary of Terms

Brihadaranyaka Upanishad	a highly advanced philosophical and mystical text, and is one of the major Upanishads
Abhyasa	Practice
Adhikari	eligible, one who is ready to learn or deserve to learn
Adhyatma	Spirituality
Adhyatmik	Spiritual person
Agni	fire or energy elements
Ajna Chakra	third eye center
Akaash	space, voidness, ether
Akashik Vijnana	astral or cosmic wisdom
Alambusha Nadi	vital energy channel connecting to the mouth
Alaya	An abode or dwelling place
Anahata Chakra	Heart center
Anandamaya Kosha	bliss body
Annamaya Kosha	Food or physical body
Antar Kumbhaka	Holding the breath in
Anu	Molecule
Apana	downward flowing subtle energy current associated with lower body areas
Apana Vayu	subtle energy current flowing downward in pelvic area, and legs
Ardha	half
Arjuna	A great warrior, son of Kunti and Pandva and disciple of Krishna
Asana	A posture, pose, state of being
Ashram	A place to learn and practice yoga and spiritual practices under guidance of Guru
Atman	Soul
Atmanubuti	self-realisation,
Bahira Kumbhaka	Holding the breath out
Bhagavad Gita	A dialogue between Krishna and Arjuna in middle of battlefield of Mahabharata on spiritual teachings and guidelines
Bhakti Yoga	Yoga of devotion
Bhokta	Consumer

Bija	seed mantras
Brahma	The creator aspect of divine in Hinduism
Brahmanda	Universe, Macrocosm
Chakra	Energy wheel
Chandogya Upanishad	a Sanskrit text embedded in the Chandogya Brahmana of the Sama Veda of Hinduism detailing meditation practices
Chandra	Lunar, Moon
Chandra Nadi Asana	Laying on right side with left side dominant for activarting chandra swara
Chandra Nadi Pranayama	Activate breathing through chandra or left nostril
Chandra Swara	Left nostril energy current
Chayopasana	Shadow gazing
Chetana	Consciousness
Chitta	Consciousness
Darshan	A view point or philosophy
Dasha Vayus	Ten subtle energy currents flowing in Nadis
Deha	Body
Dharmika Asana	devotional pose
Dharana	concentration, practice to focus our mind on single point
Dhyana	meditation, absorption of mind on single point
Drashta	Witness, viewer
Drishti	Viewpoint
Gandhari Nadi	vital energy channel connecting to the left eye
Ghatika	48 minutes
Goraksha Samhita	natha Yoga scripture composed by the great Yogī Gorakshanath
Gurkula	A home of Guru for learning yoga and Hindu spiritual practices
Guru	Spiritual teacher or guide
Hastijihva Nadi	Vital energy current connecting to the right eye
Hatha Yoga	Patha of yoga to balance Ha (solar) and Tha (Lunar) energies through asanas, mudra, pranayama, jnana yoga kriyas and shat karmas
Hatha Yoga Pradipika	A scripture composed by Swatmarama Suri in Hatha Yoga practices
Hinduism	A spiritual life style followed by Hindus based on Vedic and Upanishads teachings

Ida Nadi	The cooling, lunar energy current
Iswara Pranidhanani	Surrendering to divine, seeing life as divine blessings
Jala	water or liquid elements
Jala Neti	Nasal cleansing with saline water
Jiva	life, living being
Jnana Yoga	Yoga of Wisdom
Jnana Yoga Kriya	relaxation techniques and visualisation
Kalas	time -past, present and future
Kanda	Vital energy store in Conus Medularis
Karma	mental, verbal and physical actions
Karma Yoga	Yoga of Skill in action
Karta	Doer
Krishna	One of the incarnation of Vishnu, taught us spiritual guidelines in form of Bhagavat Gita
Krishna Paksha	waning moon period
Kriya Yoga	Yoga of action based on Tapas, Swadhyaya and Iswara Pranidhanani
Kriyas	Practices, flow, movement, action
Kuhu Nadi	vital energy channel connecting to the reproductive organs
Kumbhaka	Retention of breath
Kundalini	Latent potential vital force, resting in root chakra
Kundalini Yoga	Yoga path of Kundalini or Chakra awakening
Laya Yoga	Yoga of sound and mantra and absorption of mind in cosmic vibrations
Lokas	planes of life or consciousness
Loma	solar, positive ions of pranic vital energy
Loma Pranayama	Inhalation 6 x Hold 6 X Exhalation 6 counts, a pranayama practice
Loma Viloma Pranayama	Alternate nostril breathing
Loma Viloma Vidya	Practices to balance polarity
Maharishi Patanjali	Composer of Codifer of Raja Yoga
Manas	Mind
Mandala	A geometric energy shape
Mandala Dharna	focusing our mind on Mandala of Pancha Mahabhutas

Mandala Pranayama	Pranayama practices for Mandalas for Pancha Mahabhutas
Manipura Chakra	precious life jewel energy chakra or navel center
Manomaya Kosha	mind body
Mansika	mental
Mantra Yoga	Yoga path of mantra chanting and mediation of the essence of mantras
Mooladhara Chakra	root or foundation chakra
Mudra	A gesture or energy seal
Mukta Triveni	Liberating point of three nadis, located at third eye chakra
Nada	sound, vibrations, resonance
Nadi	subtle vital energy currents
Nadi Suddhi	Nerve or Nadi cleansing pranayama
Nasagra	Nostril
Nasagra Mudra	Pranayama gesture of hands for pranayama practices
Niyamas	Rules, observances and ethical virtues
Oli Mudras	Set of Asanas and Mudras for Kundalini Awakening
Padmasana	Lotus pose
pancha mahabhutas	Five subtle elements -prathvi, jala, vayu, agni, akaash
Pancha Tattwas	Five subtle elements -prathvi, jala, vayu, agni, akaash
Parampara	A tradition, lineage
Parmatman	Divine soul
Parvati	Wife of Lord Shiva
Pinda	Individual body, microcosm
Pingala Nadi	The heating, solar energy current
Prakriti	Nature, inherited nature
Prakriyas	Application of practices, movement, action
Pramanu	Atom
Prana	Subtle Cosmic vital force
Prana Vayu	downward flowing subtle energy current in chest, lungs, and heart
Prana Vayus	Five subtle prana energy currents
Pranamaya Kosha	Subtle energy body or sheath

Pranava	OM, cosmic vibratory sound closest to sound of divine
Pranayama	subtle vital energy work through breath as a tool
Prashna- Upanishad	It is one of the Upanishad of six main questions, asked by six seekers of truth and answered by sage Pippalapada
Prashwash	Exhalation
Prathvi	earth or solid elements
Pratyahara	sensory withdrawal
Puraka	Inhalation
Purna	complete
Purusha	Individual soul
Pusha Nadi	vital energy channel connecting to the right ear
Raja Yoga	Royal Patha of Yoga based on Patanjalis Yoga Sutras and Samkhya Yoga
Rajas	Quality of action
Rechaka	Exhalation
Rishi	Master of Spiritual Sciences
Sadhana	Sincere and disciplined practice for spiritual benefits
Sahashrara Chakra	Crown chakra
Sakshi Bhava	Witnessing awareness
Samadhi	self-realization, enlightenment, liberation
Samana Vayu	subtle energy current flowing in digestive cavity
Samaskaras	the subtle impressions of our past actions
Samayama	Inner or advance practices of Yoga based on Dharna, Dhyana and Samadhi
Samkhya	Samkhya is one of the six Darshanas of Hinduism
Samrapan	devotion and surrender
Samsthiti asana	equal standing or balanced standing pose
Sanskrita	Ancient Indian language of Gods
Satchidananda	Absolute bliss or divine joy
Sattva	Quality of pure essence.
Savitri Pranayama	a 6x3x6x3 pattern of breathing as solar pranayama
Seva	Service

Shakta	Male form of energy flowing in right side of body
Shakti	Divine creative force
Shakti	Female form of energy flowing in left side
Shankhini Nadi	vital energy channel connecting to the rectum
Shata Karmas	six cleansing practices described in hatha yoga
Shavasana	Corpse pose, relaxation pose
Shishya	Student, follower, disciple
Shiva	One of the three supreme aspects of Divine followed in Hinduism
Shiva	Cosmic transcending force
Shiva Samhita	A Yoga scripture, written as a dialogue between Lord Shiva and his wife Shakti
Shiva Swarodaya	A swara Yoga scripture, written as a dialogue between Shiva and Shakti
Shiva Swarodaya	Ancient Tantric text in Sanskrita as a dialogue between shiva and shakti
Shukla Paksha	waxing moon period
Shunyaka	Natural cessation of breath in transcendental experiences or meditation
Shusumna Nadi	balanced or central energy current
Siddha Asana	Perfect pose
Siddhis	Miracles or masteries through yoga sadhana
Soham	Mantra means 'I am Divine'
Sraddha	Faith
Sukha Asana	easy or cross legged posture
Sukha Pranayama	easy breath, equal breathing pattern of inhalation and exhalation
Sukha Purvaka Pranayama	Inhalation 6 x hold 6 x exhalation 6 x hold out 6 pattern of pranayama
Supta Vajra Asana	Reclining thunderbolt pose
Surya	Solar, Sun
Surya Bhedana	solar breathing or pranayama
Surya Nadi Asana	Laying on left side with right side dominant for activating surya swara
Surya Nadi Pranayama	Activate breathing through surya or right nostril
Surya Swara	Right nostril energy current

Sutra Neti	Nasal cleansing with cotton thread coated with bee-wax
Svayambhu-Linga	Central axis of Kundalini based at root of spine
Swa	self
Swadhisthana Chakra	sacral chakra or self-dwelling centre
Swadhyaya	Self-study, introspection
Swami	Self-realized master of yoga and self
Swara	Nostril, Energy Channel
Swara	One's own self
Swara Yoga	Patha of Yoga uses nostril breathing and ida-pingala-sushumna energy manipulations for sadhana
Swasha	Inhalation
Swasha-Prashwash	Breathing
Taittriya Upanishad	The Taittiriya Upanishad is one of the older, 'primary' Upanishads, part of the Yajur Veda. It says that the highest goal is to know the Brahman
Tamas	Quality of inertia
Tantra	energy weave, a path of yoga working on subtle energies to attain liberation
Tapas	sincere and disciplined practice for spiritual benefits
Irataka	Blink-less Gazing
Tri Gunas	three primary qualities of sattva, rajas, tamas
Udana Vayu	upward flowing energy in throat, diaphragm and excretory or expelling functions
Ujjayi	Vicrtorious pranayama
Upanishadas	Hindu scriptures on Hindu lifestyle and wisdom to attain health, peace and self-realisation
Vairajna	Non-attachment,
Vajrasana	Thunderbolt pose
Varaha-Upanishad	this is a minor Hindu text belonging to Krishna-Yajurveda
Vayu	air elements
Vedas	Four main scriptures detailing hindu life style
Vijnanamaya Kosha	cosmic wisdom body
Viloma	lunar, negative ions of pranic vital energy
Viloma Pranayama	Inhalation 6x Exhalation 6x holding the breath out 6 counts, a pranayama practice

Vishuddha Chakra	center of purity or throat chakra
Vritti	Pattern or rhythm of breathing
Vyana Vayu	subtle energy current flowing throughout the body
Yamas	Restraints or moral virtues
Yashaswini Nadi	vital energy channel connecting to the left ear
Yoga	Union, Oneness
Yoga Chudamani Upanishad	It is one of the minor Upanishads of Hinduism composed in Sanskrit, and is known as the "Crown Jewel of Yoga"
Yoga Sutras	Yoga verses of Raja Yoga composed by Maharishi Patanjali
Yogi	Masters of Yoga
Yukta Triveni	Energy store at origin or three nadis